# Advances in Cardiac Computed Tomography

*Guest Editor*

MARIO J. GARCIA, MD, FACC

# CARDIOLOGY CLINICS

www.cardiology.theclinics.com

*Consulting Editor*
MICHAEL H. CRAWFORD, MD

November 2009 • Volume 27 • Number 4

SAUNDERS an imprint of ELSEVIER, Inc.

**W.B. SAUNDERS COMPANY**
*A Division of Elsevier Inc.*

1600 John F. Kennedy Blvd. • Suite 1800 • Philadelphia, PA 19103-2899

http://www.theclinics.com

**CARDIOLOGY CLINICS Volume 27, Number 4**
**November 2009 ISSN 0733-8651, ISBN-10: 1-4377-1198-7, ISBN-13: 978-1-4377-1198-1**

Editor: Barbara Cohen-Kligerman
Developmental Editor: Theresa Collier



*Cardiology Clinics* (ISSN 0733-8651) is published quarterly by Elsevier Inc., 360 Park Avenue South, New York, NY 10010-1710. Months of issue are February, May, August, and November. Subscription prices are $244.00 per year for US individuals, $378.00 per year for US institutions, $122.00 per year for US students and residents, $298.00 per year for Canadian individuals, $470.00 per year for Canadian institutions, $346.00 per year for international individuals, $470.00 per year for international institutions and $173.00 per year for Canadian and foreign students/residents. To receive student/resident rate, orders must be accompanied by name of affiliated institution, data of term, and the *signature* of program/residency coordinator on institution letterhead. Orders will be billed at individual rate until proof of status is received. Foreign air speed delivery is included in all *Clinics* subscription prices. All prices are subject to change without notice. **POSTMASTER:** Send address changes to *Cardiology Clinics*, Elsevier Health Sciences Division, Subscription Customer Service, 3251 Riverport Lane, Maryland Heights, MO 63043. **Customer Service: 1-800-654-2452 (U.S. and Canada); 314-447-8871 (outside U.S. and Canada). Fax: 314-447-8029. E-mail: journalscustomerservice-usa@elsevier.com (for print support); journalsonlinesupport-usa@elsevier.com (for online support).**

*Reprints.* For copies of 100 or more, of articles in this publication, please contact the Commercial Reprints Department, Elsevier Inc., 360 Park Avenue South, New York, NY 10010-1710. Tel.: 212-633-3812; Fax: 212-462-1935; E-mail: reprints@elsevier.com.

*Cardiology Clinics* is also published in Spanish by McGraw-Hill Interamericana Editores S. A., P.O. Box 5-237, 06500, Mexico D. F., Mexico; in Portuguese by Reichmann and Alfonso Editores Rio de Janeiro, Brazil; and in Greek by Dimitrios P. Lagos, 8 Pondon Street, GR115-28 Ilissia, Greece.

*Cardiology Clinics* is covered in *MEDLINE/PubMed (Index Medicus), Excerpta Medica, The Cumulative Index to Nursing and Allied Health Literature* (CINAHL).

Printed in the United States of America.

# Contributors

## CONSULTING EDITOR

**MICHAEL H. CRAWFORD, MD**
Professor of Medicine, University of California, San Francisco; Lucie Stern Chair in Cardiology, and Interim Chief of Cardiology, University of California, San Francisco Medical Center, San Francisco, California

## GUEST EDITOR

**MARIO J. GARCIA, MD, FACC**
Director of Cardiovascular Imaging, Department of Medicine, The Zena and Michael Wiener Cardiovascular Institute; Professor of Medicine and Radiology, Mount Sinai Hospital and School of Medicine, New York, New York

## AUTHORS

**SUHNY ABBARA, MD**
Department of Radiology, Cardiac MR/CT Program, Cardiovascular Imaging Section, Massachusetts General Hospital, Boston, Massachusetts

**CHRISTOPH R. BECKER, MD**
Department of Clinical Radiology, Ludwig-Maximilians-University Munich, Grosshadern Clinics, Munich, Germany

**DANIEL S. BERMAN, MD**
Cedars-Sinai Medical Center, Los Angeles, California

**ANDREW R. BLUM, MD**
Department of Radiology, Cardiac MR/CT Program, Cardiovascular Imaging Section, Massachusetts General Hospital, Boston, Massachusetts

**KAVITHA M. CHINNAIYAN, MD, FACC**
Director, Cardiovascular Imaging Education, Department of Cardiology, William Beaumont Hospital, Royal Oak, Michigan

**MARIO J. GARCIA, MD, FACC**
Director of Cardiovascular Imaging, Department of Medicine, The Zena and Michael Wiener Cardiovascular Institute; Professor of Medicine and Radiology, Mount Sinai Hospital and School of Medicine, New York, New York

**JUAN GAZTANAGA, MD**
Director of Cardiac MRI/CT, Department of Medicine, Division of Cardiology, Winthrop University Hospital; Fellow, Department of Medicine, Division of Cardiology, Mount Sinai School of Medicine, New York, New York

**RICHARD T. GEORGE, MD**
Department of Medicine, Division of Cardiology, Johns Hopkins University School of Medicine, Baltimore, Maryland

**THOMAS C. GERBER, MD, PhD**
Professor of Medicine and Radiology, College of Medicine, Mayo Clinic; Consultant, Department of Radiology, Division of Cardiovascular Diseases, Mayo Clinic, Jacksonville, Florida

**JAMES A. GOLDSTEIN, MD, FACC**
Director, Research and Education, Department of Cardiology, William Beaumont Hospital, Royal Oak, Michigan

**SANDRA SIMON HALLIBURTON, PhD**
Imaging Institute, Cardiovascular Imaging, Cleveland Clinic, Cleveland, Ohio

**SUBODH B. JOSHI, MBBS**
Department of Radiology, Cardiac MR/CT Program, Cardiovascular Imaging Section, Massachusetts General Hospital, Boston, Massachusetts

**BIRGIT KANTOR, MD**
Assistant Professor of Medicine and Consultant, Division of Cardiovascular Diseases, College of Medicine, Mayo Clinic, Rochester, Minnesota

**DIVYA KAPOOR, MD**
Division of Cardiovascular Diseases, University of Missouri, Kansas City, Missouri

**YASUYUKI KOBAYASHI, MD**
Department of Medicine, Division of Cardiology, Johns Hopkins University School of Medicine, Baltimore, Maryland; St. Marianna University School of Medicine, Kawasaki, Japan

**ALBERT C. LARDO, PhD**
Departments of Medicine and Biomedical Engineering, Division of Cardiology, Johns Hopkins University School of Medicine, Baltimore, Maryland

**JOAO A.C. LIMA, MD**
Division of Cardiology, Department of Medicine and Department of Radiology, Johns Hopkins University School of Medicine, Baltimore, Maryland

**FAY Y. LIN, MD, MSc**
Department of Medicine, Division of Cardiology, Weill Medical College of Cornell University, New York Presbyterian Hospital, New York, New York

**MOUSSA MANSOUR, MD**
Department of Medicine, Section of Cardiology, Massachusetts General Hospital, Boston, Massachusetts

**CYNTHIA H. McCOLLOUGH, PhD**
Professor of Radiologic Physics and Consultant, Department of Radiology, College of Medicine, Mayo Clinic, Rochester, Minnesota

**JAMES K. MIN, MD**
Assistant Professor of Medicine and Radiology, Department of Medicine, Division of Cardiology, Weill Medical College of Cornell University, New York Presbyterian Hospital, New York, New York

**YASUO NAKAJIMA, MD, PhD**
Department of Radiology, St. Marianna University School of Medicine, Kawasaki, Japan

**GONZALO PIZARRO, MD**
Fellow, Division of Cardiology, Department of Medicine, Mount Sinai School of Medicine, New York, New York

**GILBERT L. RAFF, MD, FACC**
Director, Advanced Cardiovascular Imaging, Department of Cardiology, William Beaumont Hospital, Royal Oak, Michigan

**PAOLO RAGGI, MD**
Radiology Director, Division of Cardiology, Emory Cardiac Imaging Center; Professor of Medicine, Department of Medicine, Emory University, Atlanta, Georgia

**TOBIAS SAAM, MD**
Department of Clinical Radiology, Ludwig-Maximilians-University Munich, Grosshadern Clinics, Munich, Germany

**JAVIER SANZ, MD**
Assistant Professor, Department of Medicine, Division of Cardiology, Mount Sinai School of Medicine, New York, New York

**LESLEE J. SHAW, PhD, FASNC, FACC**
Emory University School of Medicine, Atlanta, Georgia

**RANDALL C. THOMPSON, MD**
Attending Cardiologist, Mid-America Heart Institute; Professor of Medicine, Division of Cardiovascular Diseases, University of Missouri Kansas City; Cardiovascular Consultants, Kansas City, Missouri

**SUZANNE E. ZENTKO, MD**
Department of Medicine, Division of Cardiology, Weill Medical College of Cornell University, New York Presbyterian Hospital, New York, New York

# Contents

**Foreword** xiii

Michael H. Crawford

**Preface** xv

Mario J. Garcia

**Cardiac CT: Understanding and Adopting a New Diagnostic Modality** 555

Mario J. Garcia

For many years, the holy grail in cardiac imaging was the noninvasive anatomic evaluation of the coronary arteries. Although functional tests allow for the detection of ischemia, they lack sufficient sensitivity and specificity to reliably exclude obstructive coronary artery disease in many symptomatic patients, and have practically no role in establishing the presence of non-obstructive disease in asymptomatic subjects who may benefit from preventive interventions. The very short history of cardiac CT has demonstrated rapid technological advances and the potential to eliminate the need for invasive diagnostic testing in patients who have suspected coronary artery disease. This article reviews the history of this modality, the principles and challenges for its clinical implementation, and provides a preamble to this special issue of *Cardiology Clinics*.

**Diagnostic Accuracy of CT Coronary Angiography** 563

Divya Kapoor and Randall C. Thompson

There is a rich and rapidly growing literature on the diagnostic utility of coronary CT angiography (CTA) and its performance relative to other modalities such as stress testing and invasive coronary angiography. Earlier studies of 16-slice coronary CTA showed wide variability in sensitivity (30%–95%) and some variability in specificity (86%–98%). With 40- and 64-slice coronary CTA, more of the chest is covered with each spin of the gantry, the breath hold is shorter, and there are fewer uninterpretable segments than with 16-slice coronary CTA. The very high negative predictive value is especially helpful in ruling out coronary artery disease in patients who have low to intermediate pretest likelihood of CAD.

**The Prognostic Value of Cardiac Computed Tomographic Angiography** 573

Fay Y. Lin, Suzanne E. Zentko, and James K. Min

With advancements in temporal and spatial resolution, CT has excellent diagnostic characteristics for non-invasive evaluation of coronary artery disease in appropriate patients. Nevertheless, clinical usefulness of diagnostic testing requires not only high diagnostic accuracy but also risk stratification for patient management. Current guidelines for risk stratification of patients with coronary artery disease rely primarily upon functional testing; alternatively, anatomic risk stratification may also be performed with invasive coronary angiography. This article reviews current and emerging concepts in the prognostic value of cardiac CT angiography.

**Cardiac CT in the Emergency Department** 587

Kavitha M. Chinnaiyan, Gilbert L. Raff, and James A. Goldstein

In the United States alone, nearly 6 million patients present annually to emergency departments with complaints of chest pain suggestive of acute coronary ischemia. Most of these patients have a non-negligible risk for acute coronary syndrome(s) (ACS) and undergo extended observation and workup for an ischemic cause. Of those admitted for extended observation, less than 30% of patients have true ACS. In patients with a low to intermediate probability, cardiac CT performs well in ruling out coronary artery disease, and American College of Cardiology and American Heart Association guidelines deem this application to be "appropriate." This article reviews the application of CT for the evaluation of acute chest pain the emergency department.

**Functional Versus Anatomic Imaging in Patients with Suspected Coronary Artery Disease** 597

Leslee J. Shaw and Daniel S. Berman

Patients with suspected or known coronary artery disease often require evaluation by cardiac imaging tests. The purpose of these tests may vary according to each individual patient, from establishing or ruling out obstructive coronary artery disease as the cause of symptoms to determining the risk of future cardiac events and guiding the selection of medical therapy and revascularization. With the adoption of cardiac CT, most patients can have a complete evaluation noninvasively. The challenge is to determine when anatomical evaluation of coronary artery disease or functional evaluation of the burden of ischemia may be required. This article reviews the relative value of anatomical versus functional imaging and their complementary role in different clinical scenarios.

**Cardiac CT in Asymptomatic Patients at Risk** 605

Paolo Raggi

Atherosclerosis is a systemic process that can develop as early as the second or third decade of life. A significant percentage of patients who experience acute coronary syndromes often have non-obstructive coronary artery disease and thus cannot be diagnosed by their symptoms or conventional functional stress testing. It has been proposed that early detection of atherosclerosis would generate novel opportunities for primary prevention through changes in lifestyle or even through drug therapy, especially in patients at high cardiovascular risk. Calcium scoring is a simple, reproducible, and widely available test that has been extensively validated over the past two decades. In this article, the utility of calcium scoring and the potential application of CT coronary angiography in asymptomatic patients at risk are reviewed.

**Evaluation of Coronary Atherosclerotic Plaques** 611

Christoph R. Becker and Tobias Saam

In many patients, unheralded myocardial infarction associated with a mortality of approximately 20% is the first manifestation of coronary artery disease. Approximately 40% of the population is considered to have a moderate midterm risk of 10% to 20%. Any of the stratification schemes suffers from a lack of accuracy to correctly determine the risk, and uncertainty exists regarding how to treat individuals who have been identified to be at intermediate risk. Other tools providing information about the necessity to reassure or to treat these patients are warranted. Currently, the assessment of the atherosclerotic plaque burden by CT may be able provide valid information for this cohort. This article discusses the potential value and limitations of cardiac CT for evaluating coronary atherosclerotic plaque.

**CT Applications in Electrophysiology** **619**

Subodh B. Joshi, Andrew R. Blum, Moussa Mansour, and Suhny Abbara

In recent years, extraordinary advances have been made in the management of cardiac arrhythmias. Increasingly complex procedures are being performed, and the breadth of conditions for which invasive arrhythmia therapy is indicated continues to grow. In addition to atrial and ventricular ablation procedures for treating arrhythmias, implantable defibrillators and biventricular pacemakers for cardiac resynchronization therapy have made electrophysiology an important part of heart failure management.

**Evaluation of Cardiac Valves Using Multi-Detector CT** **633**

Juan Gaztanaga, Gonzalo Pizarro, and Javier Sanz

Cardiac CT is an accurate and reasonable alternative modality for valvular imaging. It is used primarily for the evaluation of coronary artery disease; however, important information regarding valvular anatomy and function can be derived from CT. Calcification is a common CT finding in various valvular abnormalities and carries important diagnostic and prognostic value. In addition, valvular morphology, stenosis, and regurgitation also are detected on contrast enhanced scans, with good correlation with trans-thoracic echocardiography and other techniques.

**Left Ventricular Function, Myocardial Perfusion and Viability** **645**

Yasuyuki Kobayashi, Albert C. Lardo, Yasuo Nakajima, Joao A.C. Lima, and Richard T. George

Cardiac computed tomography is now poised to revolutionize the practice of cardiology. Multi-detector row CT (MDCT) has the potential to evaluate cardiac function, myocardial perfusion, and viability. These capabilities, combined with the robust ability of MDCT to noninvasively image the coronary arteries, makes MDCT a comprehensive tool for the evaluation of coronary artery disease and its anatomic and physiologic impact on the myocardium. Recent technologic advances in MDCT technology in regards to detector coverage, and spatial and temporal resolution promise to improve the capabilities of cardiac CT in the assessment of cardiac function, perfusion, and viability.

**Recent Technologic Advances in Multi-Detector Row Cardiac CT** **655**

Sandra Simon Halliburton

Recent technical advances in multi-detector row CT have resulted in lower radiation dose, improved temporal and spatial resolution, decreased scan time, and improved tissue differentiation. Lower radiation doses have resulted from the use of pre-patient *z* collimators, the availability of thin-slice axial data acquisition, the increased efficiency of ECG-based tube current modulation, and the implementation of iterative reconstruction algorithms. Faster gantry rotation and the simultaneous use of two x-ray sources have led to improvements in temporal resolution, and gains in spatial resolution have been achieved through application

# Cardiology Clinics

## FORTHCOMING ISSUES

*February 2010*

**Advanced Applied Interventional Cardiology**
Samin Sharma, MD, and
Annapoorna Kini, MD,
*Guest Editors*

*May 2010*

**Controversies in Thoracic Aortic Disease**
John Elefteriades, MD,
*Guest Editor*

*August 2010*

**Diabetes, the Kidney and Cardiovascular Risk**
George Bakris, MD, FASN,
*Guest Editor*

## RECENT ISSUES

*August 2009*

**Advances in Coronary Angiography**
S. James Chen, PhD, and
John D. Carroll, MD,
*Guest Editors*

*May 2009*

**Nuclear Cardiology—From Perfusion to Tissue Biology**
Frank Bengel, MD,
*Guest Editor*

*February 2009*

**Atrial Fibrillation**
Ranjan K. Thakur, MD, MPH, FHRS, and
Andrea Natale, MD, FACC, FHRS,
*Guest Editors*

## ISSUES OF RELATED INTEREST

*Heart Failure Clinics,* October 2009 (Vol. 5, No. 4)
**Biomarkers in Heart Failure**
Eugene Braunwald, MD, *Guest Editor*
Available at: http://www.heartfailure.theclinics.com/

*Heart Failure Clinics,* July 2009 (Vol. 5, No. 3)
**Cardiovascular Magnetic Resonance in Heart Failure**
Raymond J. Kim, MD, and Dudley J. Pennell, MD, FRCP, FACC, *Guest Editors*
Available at: http://www.heartfailure.theclinics.com/

# Foreword

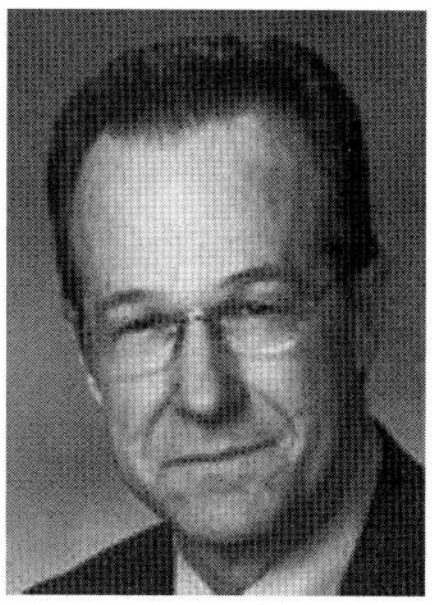

Michael H. Crawford, MD
*Consulting Editor*

The November 2003 issue of *Cardiology Clinics* was devoted to cardiac computed tomography (CT). In the intervening 6 years tremendous advances in this technology have occurred. We now can legitimately claim that computed tomography angiography (CTA) of the coronary arteries is available. In the evaluation of patients with suspected coronary artery disease, many guidelines consider CTA an alternative to stress testing. In the typical patient with exercise-induced symptoms, stress imaging still makes sense, but there are many other patients in whom CTA may be preferable. For example, we are using it frequently in pre–noncardiac organ transplant patients to exclude significant coronary artery disease (CAD) before committing a scarce resource (organ) to a patient.

The use of CTA in primary prevention patients is more controversial, because the Bayes theorem becomes important in considering diagnostic test interpretation in populations with a low prevalence of disease. Also, given our current armamentarium for preventing CAD, it is difficult to prove that CTA information changes outcomes. However, it is clear that CTA information motivates physicians to be more aggressive therapeutically.

Cardiac CT has other uses that are also discussed in this issue, such as atherosclerotic plaque characterization, myocardial perfusion and viability, heart valve function and anatomic imaging for electrophysiology studies, and ablations. These topics and all the particulars the clinician needs to know about cardiac CT are covered in this excellent issue edited by Dr. Mario Garcia. He has assembled an internationally known group of experts to bring us up to date in this rapidly emerging field. This issue is full of important information that every cardiologist needs to know.

Michael H. Crawford, MD
Division of Cardiology
Department of Medicine
University of California
San Francisco Medical Center
505 Parnassus Avenue, Box 0124
San Francisco, CA 94143-0124, USA

E-mail address:
crawfordm@medicine.ucsf.edu



Cardiol Clin 27 (2009) xiii
doi:10.1016/j.ccl.2009.07.001

# Preface

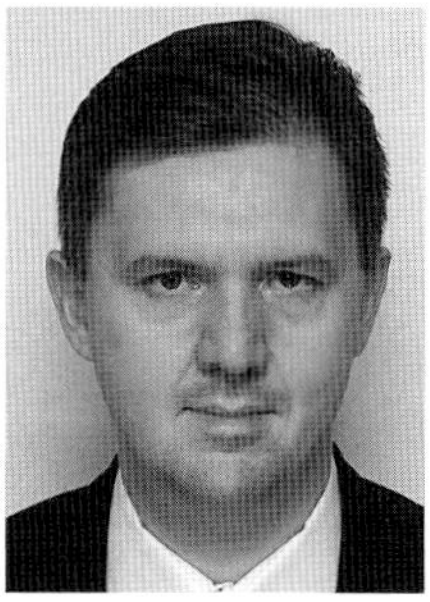

Mario J. Garcia, MD, FACC
*Guest Editor*

Patients with known or suspected coronary artery disease who are asymptomatic or who have stable symptoms are often evaluated noninvasively. Functional tests, such as stress electrocardiography, stress echocardiography, or stress nuclear perfusion imaging, detect and quantify the presence of ischemia based on electrical, mechanical, or perfusion abnormalities, indirectly establishing the burden of coronary artery disease. Although these tests have been shown to provide important prognostic information including the prediction of benefit from revascularization, they have limited accuracy for establishing or excluding the diagnosis of obstructive coronary artery disease.

More recently, multidetector CT has emerged as a tool to evaluate noninvasively the coronary anatomy. Multidetector CT has overcome many of its original limitations and now provides ECG-gated acquisition with short acquisition time, submillimeter spatial resolution, and adequate temporal resolution, allowing excellent visualization of the coronary arteries. Over the last 10 years, the rate of technologic advancements leading to improved coronary angiography with multidetector CT has rapidly exceeded those of other cardiac imaging modalities. Image quality is undergoing constant refinement, and the number of uninterpretable coronary studies has gradually decreased from 20% to 40% using four-detector, to 15% to 25% with 16-detector, and is now as low as 3% to 10% with 64-detector systems. Although CT coronary angiography has demonstrated higher sensitivity for the detection of coronary artery disease than any other noninvasive imaging modality, many experts still question the clinical use and safety of CT coronary angiography, raising considerable debate in the medical community.

This issue of *Cardiology Clinics* includes a series of articles that provide a state-of-the-art summary of the current clinical applications of cardiac CT, reviews data that support the accuracy and the prognostic use of CT coronary angiography, and reports on the newest technologic advances and promising future applications of this exciting imaging modality.

Readers of *Cardiology Clinics* will enjoy this issue and will find the information and expert opinions very useful to their clinical practice.

Mario J. Garcia, MD, FACC
The Zena and Michael Wiener
Cardiovascular Institute
Mount Sinai Hospital and School of Medicine
One Gustave Levy Place
New York, NY 10029, USA

E-mail address:
Mario.garcia@mountsinai.org (M.J. Garcia)

Cardiol Clin 27 (2009) xv
doi:10.1016/j.ccl.2009.06.014

# Cardiac CT: Understanding and Adopting a New Diagnostic Modality

Mario J. Garcia, MD, FACC

**KEYWORDS**

- Computed tomography • Coronary angiography
- Coronary artery disease • Atherosclerosis
- Cardiac imaging

Coronary artery disease (CAD) is the leading cause of death in the western world and the leading cause of premature permanent disability.[1] Invasive coronary angiography is considered the diagnostic standard for establishing the presence and severity of significant CAD; however, revascularization is required in less than 50% of patients undergoing diagnostic coronary angiography. As invasive catheterization procedures have associated mortality (0.15%) and morbidity (1.5%),[2] attention has been turned to finding alternative noninvasive diagnostic tests.

Noninvasive imaging testing for detecting CAD has evolved significantly over the last 50 years. For many years, it has been known that the symptoms of CAD depend upon the balance of myocardial oxygen supply and oxygen demand. During stress, myocardial oxygen demand increases, but myocardial blood flow cannot increase any further, leading to the development of ischemia. Myocardial ischemia results in progressive metabolic and functional alterations, including reduced relative perfusion, abnormal regional diastolic and systolic myocardial function, and electrical repolarization abnormalities. On these principles, different stress testing modalities attempt to indirectly establish the diagnosis of obstructive CAD by identifying one or several of these sequelae. In clinical practice, however, the accuracy of stress imaging tests is less than 85% for detecting obstructive disease and negligible for detecting non-obstructive CAD.[3] The reported sensitivity for exercise echocardiography ranges from 71% to 97%, and the specificity ranges from 64% to over 90%. The average reported sensitivity and specificity for exercise Single photon emission computed tomography (SPECT) are 86% and 74%, respectively.[4] This represents a significant limitation, because many acute coronary syndromes occur in patients who were previously asymptomatic and had nonobstructive CAD. In theory, anatomic imaging of the coronaries could identify these patients.

From its inception, there was a desire to apply the technology of radiographic CT to imaging of the cardiovascular system because of the potential for acquiring cross-sectional images, differentiating soft tissue, and quantifying structural and functional parameters. Cardiac imaging with CT, however, requires:

- High temporal resolution to limit cardiac motion artifacts
- High spatial resolution to visualize small cardiac anatomic details
- Fast anatomic coverage allowing scanning of the heart during a breath hold to reduce respiratory motion artifacts
- Synchronization of data acquisition or reconstruction to the cardiac cycle to ensure imaging during a desired cardiac phase

In the late 1980s helical or spiral scanning was adopted in CT. In this mode, data began to be acquired during continuous rotation of the gantry

Department of Medicine, The Zena and Michael Wiener Cardiovascular Institute, Mount Sinai Hospital and School of Medicine, One Gustave Levy Place, NY 10029, USA
*E-mail address:* mario.garcia@mountsinai.org

Cardiol Clin 27 (2009) 555–562
doi:10.1016/j.ccl.2009.06.008
0733-8651/09/$ – see front matter 

and continuous movement of the patient table,[5] thereby reducing acquisition time. The availability of simultaneous multidetector acquisition with subsecond rotation times and ECG-synchronized scanning in the late 1990s brought helical CT into the domain of cardiac imaging.[6] Multidetector CT (MDCT) technology gradually overcame many of its initial limitations, and now can provide ECG-gated acquisition with short acquisition time, submillimeter spatial resolution, and adequate spatial resolution (80 to 220 milliseconds), thus allowing excellent visualization of the coronary arteries. Moreover, the rate of technological advancements leading to improved coronary angiography with MDCT has exceeded those of other noninvasive imaging modalities. Noncontrast ECG-gated MDCT scans provide accurate and reproducible measurement of coronary calcification, which carries important prognostic indications. With the injection of contrast, a three-dimensional coronary angiogram (CTA) may be obtained that includes not only visualization of the coronary lumen, but also the presence, extent, and location of calcified and noncalcified atherosclerotic plaques.

Although the actual acquisition of CTA studies takes less than 15 seconds, patient preparation and data interpretation require extensive training and extreme attention to detail. Even in expert hands, the average time required for interpretation exceeds by far the time required for interpretation of nuclear perfusion or echocardiographic studies. A description of the steps required for patient preparation, performance of the scan, and interpretation follows.

## PERFORMING A CARDIAC CT

### *Patient Preparation and Data Acquisition*

At the time of scheduling, a brief review of the medical history and indications for the procedure is performed, including existing relative or absolute contraindications for the use of iodine contrast, renal function, and patient's heart rate and rhythm. A stable, low heart rate is required at the time of the procedure, because motion artifacts can occur, given current limitations in temporal resolution of existing scanners. Oral (metoprolol or atenolol, 50 to 100 mg) or intravenous (metoprolol, 5 to 30 mg) beta-blockers administered before the study are used to obtain ideally a resting heart rate below 60 beats per minute. Beta-blockers reduce heart rate variability during the scan, and for that reason, their administration is recommended almost routinely unless contraindicated.

Because high intravenous contrast injection rates are required to attain adequate vessel opacification, a large bore intravenous catheter should be secured in the antecubital veins and adequately tested to minimize the risk of infiltration. After the intravenous catheter is inserted, the patient is positioned supine in the CT table, and ECG leads are positioned in the chest or abdomen. A careful and detailed explanation of the procedure is important, because image quality largely depends on patient's compliance.

Once adequate ECG triggering is confirmed, data acquisition is started. A survey scan (planar radiograph mode), is performed first to select the region of interest (from the carina to slightly below the diaphragm). The timing and duration of contrast administration are predetermined using a test bolus or directly triggering acquisition after the initial appearance of contrast in the ascending or descending aorta.

### *Image Processing and Interpretation*

CTA provides complex and detailed three-dimensional data sets, which are reconstructed from the raw data file, according to specific phases of the cardiac cycles. In most patients who have a heart rate below 70 beats per minute, the best phase free of motion is centered on 75% of the RR interval, corresponding to the diastasis phase of diastole. At higher rates, diastasis disappears; therefore image reconstruction at about 50% of the cardiac cycle (isovolumic relaxation) is preferred. Nevertheless, there is significant patient-to-patient variability, and often several phases reconstructed at 5% to 10% intervals need to be examined.

Once the best phase for analysis is determined, careful examination of each vessel is performed from three-dimensional derived multiplanar reconstructed images. Careful adjustment of image contrast and window levels is done to differentiate the iodine-enhanced lumen from calcified and noncalcified plaques. This procedure is repeated for each vessel segment and its branches.

## APPLICATIONS

### *Detection of Coronary Artery Stenosis*

**Figs. 1** and **2** demonstrate volume rendered and curved multiplanar reformatted (MPR) views of a normal and a severely stenosed right coronary artery. The first single center studies investigated the accuracy of 16-row CTA for detecting coronary artery stenosis in patients who had known or suspected CAD referred for invasive coronary angiography.[7,8] In all these studies, analysis of the CTA data was performed by investigators blinded to the results of invasive angiography, and in many, it was limited to coronary segments of more than

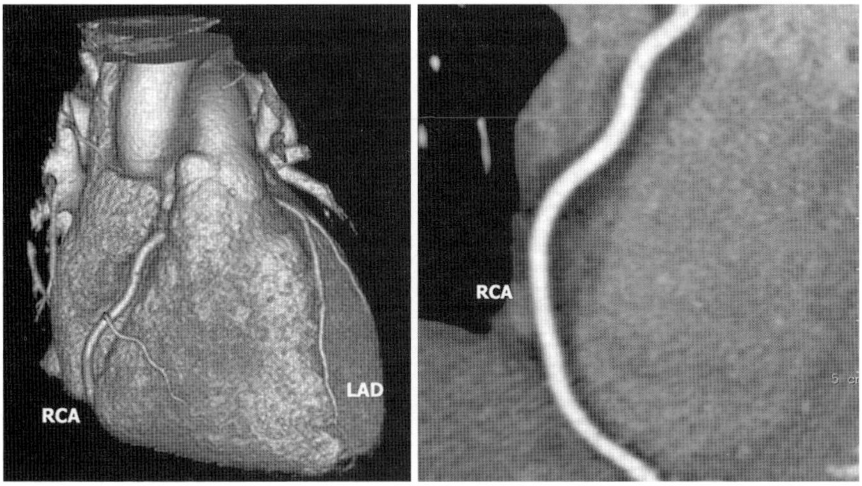


**Fig. 1.** Volume rendered (*left*) and curved multiplanar reformatted (MPR, *right*) views of a normal right coronary artery (RCA).

1.5 or 2 mm in diameter. In most cases, significant coronary artery stenosis was defined as at least 50% diameter reduction, to define sensitivity, specificity, and positive and negative predictive values. The prevalence of significant CAD in patients enrolled in these studies was 53% to 83%. Based on these studies, the sensitivity of CTA ranged between 72% and 95% per coronary segment, and 85% to 100% when using each patient as the denominator unit. The specificity per segment was reported between 86% and 98% and between 78% and 86% per patient. Positive predictive values have ranged between 72% and 90% per segment and 81% and 97% per patient, and negative predictive values have ranged between 97% and 99% and 82% and 100%, respectively. As expected, sensitivity has been higher in those studies that excluded segments with a diameter less than 1.5 mm. Most experts agree that the ability of detecting obstructive coronary disease in smaller-caliber vessels is less important, because myocardial revascularization often is not required or it is unable to be performed.

In a multicenter trial that studied the accuracy of CTA in 187 patients referred for diagnostic invasive angiography, the sensitivity, specificity, and positive and negative predictive values for detecting more than 50% luminal stenoses were 89%, 65%, 13%, and 99%.[9] In this study, nonevaluable segments were censored as positive, because in clinical practice they also would lead to performance of angiography. The sensitivity, specificity, and positive and negative predictive values for detecting subjects

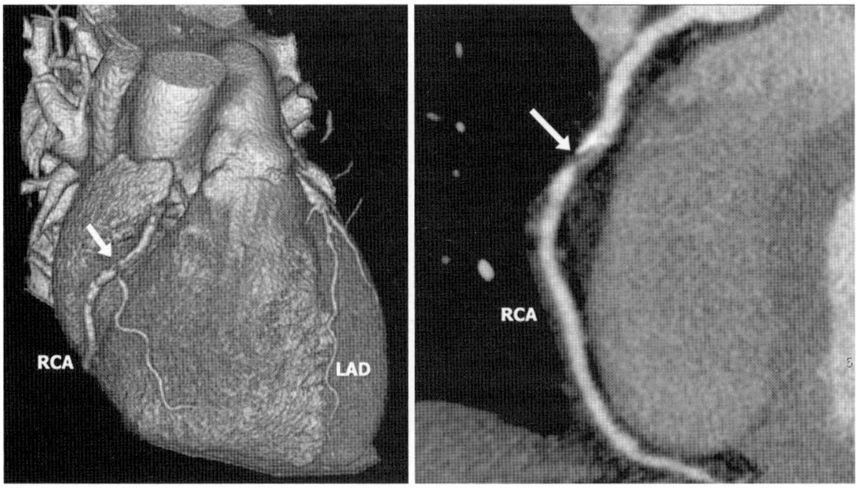


**Fig. 2.** Volume rendered (*left*) and curved multiplanar reformatted (MPR, *right*) views of a severely stenosed right coronary artery (RCA).

with at least one positive segment were 98%, 54%, 50%, and 99%. The high negative predictive value indicated that if applied in selected patients who had low–intermediate prevalence of CAD, the test would be useful to exclude CAD as the cause of chest pain. This recently was demonstrated in a study that compared the performance characteristics of CT coronary angiography in patients who had low, intermediate, and high expected prevalence of CAD.[10]

On the other hand, the high number of nonevaluable and false-positive segments suggests that CT coronary angiography performed with 16-row MDCT may lead to overdiagnosis if applied to patients who have high probability or already established CAD. The assessment of coronary artery stenosis in patients who have extensive coronary calcification is challenging. The actual volume of calcified plaques tends to be overestimated, leading to underestimation of the coronary lumen size. In a study that analyzed the performance of CTA after excluding patients who had a calcium score less than 1000, sensitivity and specificity were 98% and 98% when only those patients who had a score were included ($n$ = 46), compared with 77% and 97% for all patients ($n$ = 60).[11] Because symptomatic patients who have very high calcium scores have a very high probability of having obstructive CAD, it is reasonable to avoid CT angiography and proceed directly to invasive catheterization in these patients.

The new generation of 64-slice MDCT systems provides greater coverage per rotation, allowing shorter breath holds and higher contrast injection rates, thus reducing artifacts related to patient breath hold compliance and heart rate variability.[12–14] The superior spatial and temporal resolution of 64-slice MDCT has led to measurable improvement in image quality.[15] In several single and multicenter studies, the sensitivities and specificities for the detection of coronary artery stenosis have been reported between 92% and 95% and 95% and 99%, respectively. The number of nonevaluable segments excluded has been reduced below 10%,[16–18] also representing a significant improvement when compared with previous-generation scanners. A comprehensive review of the accuracy and performance characteristics of CT coronary angiography for diagnosing obstructive CAD is available in the article by Thompson in this issue.

## *Evaluation of Atherosclerotic Plaque Morphology*

**Fig. 3** shows a multiplanar reconstructed image of a severely stenosed left anterior descending artery with both calcified and noncalcified plaques. Until recently, intravascular ultrasound (IVUS) was the only diagnostic tool capable of detecting the presence, extent, and composition of these plaques in the coronary arteries in vivo.[19–21] Unfortunately, the wide application of IVUS as a screening tool for risk assessment is impractical because of the need for and high cost of invasive catheterization. In contrast to invasive coronary angiography, CTA is also capable of imaging the vessel wall. Recent studies have documented the ability of CTA to visualize atherosclerotic coronary plaques[22–25] and differentiate calcified from noncalcified lesions based on Hounsfield unit values. In a series of 22 patients clinically referred for IVUS, CTA correctly identified the presence of coronary atherosclerotic plaques in 41 of 50 affected segments.[25] Whether CTA could be used in clinical practice as a screening test remains to be proven, but in selected patients at low–intermediate risk, it could help to justify lifelong aggressive preventive intervention. CTA plaque characterization also could serve to devise optimal revascularization strategies. A detailed review of the application of CT for atherosclerotic plaque assessment is provided in the article by Becker in this issue.

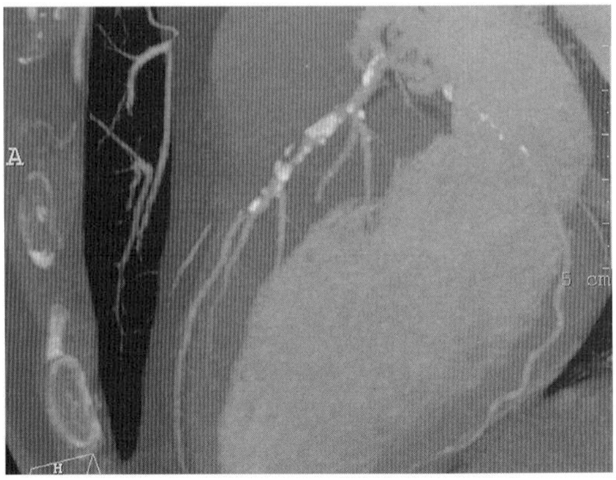

**Fig. 3.** Multiplanar reconstructed image of a severely stenosed left anterior descending artery with both calcified and noncalcified plaques.

## *Other Clinical Applications*

Presently, with the use of pulmonary vein isolation procedures for atrial fibrillation, MDCT allows:

- Evaluation of the left atrial, pulmonary vein anatomy and establishment of the anatomic position of the esophagus to avoid its perforation during the procedure
- Detection of pulmonary vein stenosis following the procedure, which varies according to the experience of the operator

and the technique, but may be as high as 20% as detected by cardiac CT[26]

This modality has high sensitivity for detecting left atrial appendage thrombi, but reduced specificity, as it is often difficult to differentiate reduced opacification because of slow flow versus actual presence of a thrombus. A detailed review of the applications of CT in electrophysiology is available in the article by Abbara in this issue.

Cardiac CT is a useful imaging modality for evaluating cardiac masses, particularly to determine their location, extent, and anatomic relationships.[27] Cardiac CT (CCT) provides superior resolution for detecting calcification and evaluating perfusion and relationship to noncardiac structures. CCT may determine pericardial thickness and tissue characteristics accurately.

## IMPLEMENTATION OF CT CORONARY ANGIOGRAPHY IN CLINICAL PRACTICE

Given the recent adoption of this technology, evidence to support improved clinical outcomes or reduced costs is lacking. One must recognize that these data will become available over time, with its increased clinical use. Historically, nuclear scintigraphy and stress echocardiography were adopted several years before evidence became available to support their outcome benefit. Nevertheless, the impact of implementing CTA in clinical practice can be predicted, taking into account the performance characteristics of CTA compared with current noninvasive imaging modalities.

**Fig. 4** compares the false-negative rates of both tests according to disease prevalence and based on sensitivities and specificities published in the literature. In patients who have low probability of obstructive CAD (eg, 10%), the number of missed cases is low for both modalities. Exercise nuclear scintigraphy will miss 12 cases per 1000 patients who have obstructive CAD (1.2%), whereas CTA will miss 4 cases per 1000 patients (0.4%). In patients who have intermediate risk (eg, 50%), however, the number of missed cases is significantly lower for CTA. Exercise nuclear scintigraphy will miss 60 cases per 1000 patients who have obstructive CAD (6%), whereas CTA will miss 20 cases per 1000 patients (2%).

**Fig. 5** compares the false-positive rates of both tests according to disease prevalence. In patients who have low probability of obstructive CAD (eg, 10%), the number of cases overdiagnosed as positive is significantly lower for CTA. Exercise nuclear scintigraphy will overdiagnose 261 cases per 1000 patients without obstructive CAD (26%), whereas CTA will overdiagnose only 126 cases per 1000 patients (1.2%). In patients who have intermediate risk (eg, 50%), the number of overdiagnosed cases is significantly lower for both modalities. Exercise nuclear scintigraphy will overdiagnose 145 cases per 1000 patients without obstructive CAD (14%), whereas CTA will overdiagnose 70 cases per 1000 patients (7%). A detailed analysis of the diagnostic accuracy of stress testing versus CTA is provided in the article by Berman in this issue.

Accordingly, in patients who have lower probability of obstructive CAD, CTA used as a primary evaluation tool may reduce the number of false-positive cases significantly, therefore reducing the need for unnecessary downstream testing including conventional angiography. In patients who have moderate probability, CTA may reduce the rate of false-negative cases. Finally, in

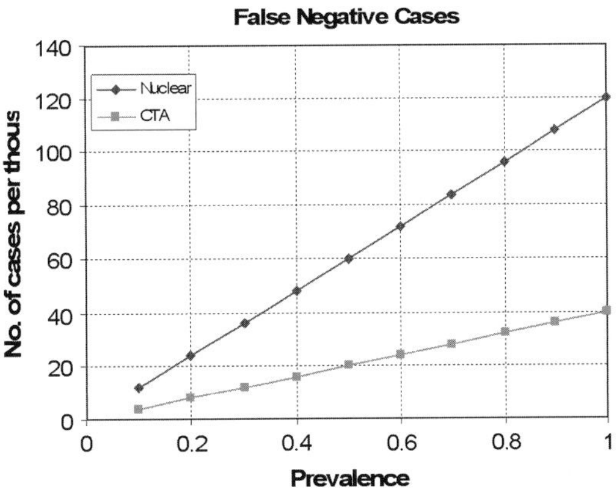


**Fig. 4.** Comparison of false-negative rates of coronary angiogram (CTA) and SPECT stress myocardial perfusion imaging SPECT according to disease prevalence and averaged reported sensitivities and specificities for both tests.

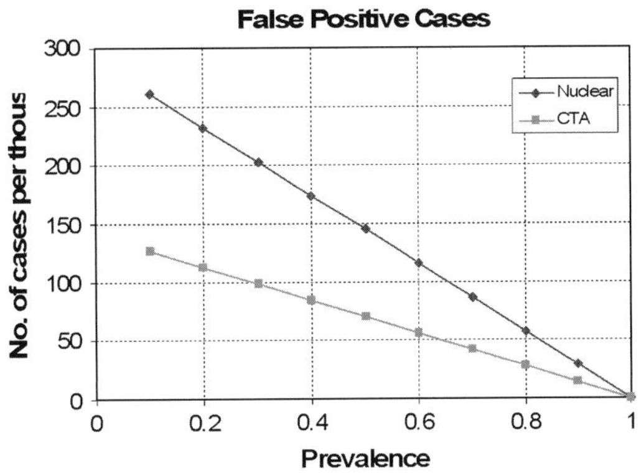


**Fig. 5.** Comparison of false positive rates of coronary angiogram (CTA) and SPECT stress myocardial perfusion imaging SPECT according to disease prevalence and averaged reported sensitivities and specificities for both tests.

selected equivocal cases, CTA and stress testing could be employed as complementary modalities (**Fig. 6**).

It is important to consider, nevertheless, that these assumptions have not been tested prospectively in randomized clinical trials. Furthermore, functional (stress) tests provide important prognostic information and help to identify which patients are more likely to derive benefit from revascularization. Several studies have shown that a normal exercise stress study predicts a very low likelihood (less than 1%) of adverse events such as cardiac death or myocardial infarction for at least 12 months and that this level of risk is independent of gender, age, symptom status, and even presence of anatomic coronary artery disease. In those patients who have abnormal scans, baseline clinical characteristics, such as diabetes, and the extent and severity of perfusion abnormalities permit one to define incremental levels of risk, and which populations of patients will benefit most from revascularization.[28] Prognostic data with cardiac CT are emerging. A comprehensive review of these data are provided in the article by Min within this issue.

## THE FUTURE OF CARDIAC CT

The most important future goals in cardiac CT will be:

- To improve accuracy in technically difficult cases
- To reduce radiation exposure
- To ensure quality standards for performance and interpretation
- To refine appropriate indications validated by outcome studies

Since the introduction of four-row MDCT scanners, gantry speed has increased from 500 milliseconds per revolution to close to 300 milliseconds. With dual-source systems, a second set of radiograph tubes and collimation systems is placed at 90°.[29] Both detectors allow for the simultaneous acquisition of 64 overlapping 0.6 mm slices by means of double z-sampling. Temporal resolution is equivalent to 25% of the rotation time plus the fan angle, slightly below 100 milliseconds. A recent study performed in 100 patients with a mean heart rate of 68 plus 11 beats per minute demonstrated a per-patient sensitivity and specificity of 99% and 87%, respectively, without administration of beta-blockers.[30]

Increased z-coverage per rotation has been proposed as a means of reducing radiation and limiting respiratory motion reconstruction artifacts. A typical acquisition with a four-row MDCT scanner required 30 to 40 seconds breath hold for a cardiac study, compared with the 6 to 8 second breath hold required for a study performed with a 64-row system. Newly introduced 256- and 320-row MDCT systems use a wide-area cylindrical two-dimensional detector incorporating present CT technology mounted on the gantry frame of a 16-row MDCT.[31] Total radiation exposure may be reduced by 50% compared with a similar configuration 64-row MDCT system, given the lower required acquisition time.[32] A detailed overview of recent technological advances in cardiac CT is provided in the article by Halliburton in this issue.

Current strategies to minimize radiation include imaging with lower tube voltage (100 kVp) and prospective ECG-triggered acquisition. In the standard retrospective gated acquisition, images are obtained during continuous advancement of the table through the gantry, thus generating a spiral or helical volume of data. In the newly implemented prospective triggered acquisition, the

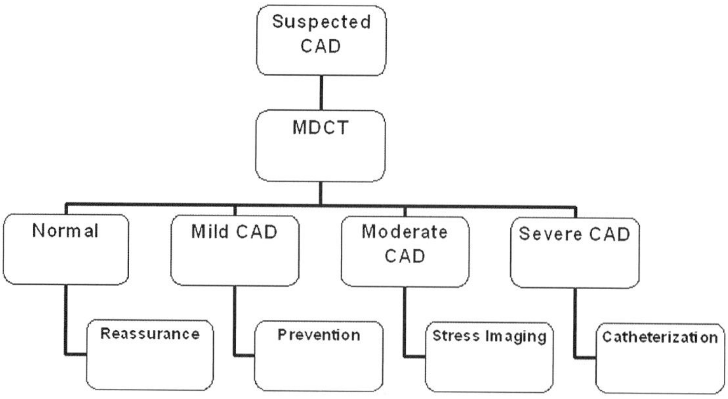


**Fig. 6.** Expected outcomes after a cardiac CT and potential complementary role of stress imaging.

table is advanced a distant equivalent to the width of the detector panel and then stopped. The radiograph tube then is turned on at the chosen phase of the cardiac cycle for one-half gantry rotation and turned off. The table is advanced again, and the process is repeated until complete volume coverage is obtained. This method has the potential to reduce radiation exposure significantly, because radiographs are administered only during a small portion of the cardiac cycle. In a recent study, image quality and patient radiation dose were compared in patients who underwent 64-detector CT coronary angiography performed with prospective ECG gating and patients matched for clinical features who underwent 64-detector CT coronary angiography performed with retrospective ECG gating.[33] The number of coronary artery segments that could not be evaluated in each group was similar (1.1% (7 of 614) in the prospective group versus 1.5% (10 of 647) in the retrospective group, $P = .53$). In this study, mean patient radiation dose was 77% lower for prospective gating (4.2 mSv) than for retrospective gating (18.1 mSv) ($P<.01$).

## SUMMARY

Given the recent adoption of MDCT technology, evidence to support improved clinical outcomes or reduced costs is limited. One must recognize that outcome data will become available over time, with increased clinical use. Meanwhile, the high negative predictive value of this test makes it ideal for establishing or excluding CAD in patients who have low–intermediate probability. When used as a primary test, a normal CTA study virtually excludes the presence of CAD. CTA studies that demonstrate the presence of atherosclerotic plaque without significant luminal stenosis may be useful to establish the need for implementing secondary prevention, although outcome data are lacking to support clinical utility of this strategy. Functional testing should follow CTA studies that show moderate–severe stenosis in most cases, given the high prevalence of false-positive CTA results. In patients who have nondiagnostic, equivocal, or unexpected functional stress test results, CTA also may be useful as a confirmatory test, therefore reducing the need for diagnostic coronary angiography.

## REFERENCES


1. American Heart Association, American Stroke Association. Heart and stroke statistical update. Dallas (TX): The American Heart Association; 2002.
2. Kennedy JW. Complications associated with cardiac catheterization and angiography. Cathet Cardiovasc Diagn 1982;8:5–11.
3. Gibbons RJ, Balady GJ, Beasley JW, et al. ACC/AHA guidelines for exercise testing. A report of the American College of Cardiology/American Heart Association Task Force on Practice Guidelines (Committee on Exercise Testing). J Am Coll Cardiol 1997;30(1):260–311.
4. Underwood SR, Anagnostopoulos C, Cerqueira M, et al. Myocardial perfusion scintigraphy: the evidence. Eur J Nucl Med Mol Imaging 2004;31:261–91.
5. Crawford CR, King KF. Computed tomography scanning with simultaneous patient translation. Med Phys 1990;17(6):967–82.
6. Hu H, He HD, Foley WD, et al. Four multidectector-row helical CT: image quality and volume coverage speed. Radiology 2000;215:55–62.
7. d'Othee BJanne, Siebert U, Cury R, et al. A systematic review on diagnostic accuracy of CT-based detection of significant coronary artery disease. Eur J Radiol 2008;65(3):449–61.
8. Gopalakrishnan P, Wilson GT, Tak T. Accuracy of multislice computed tomography coronary angiography: a pooled estimate. Cardiol Rev 2008;16(4):189–96.
9. Garcia MJ, Lessick J, Hoffmann MHK. Accuracy of 16-row multidetector computed tomography for the assessment of coronary artery stenosis. JAMA 2006;296:404–11.
10. Meijboom WB, van Mieghem CA, Mollet NR, et al. 64-slice computed tomography coronary angiography in patients with high, intermediate, or low pretest probability of significant coronary artery disease. J Am Coll Cardiol 2007;50:1469–75.
11. Kuettner A, Trabold T, Schroeder S, et al. Noninvasive detection of coronary lesions using 16-detector multislice spiral computed tomography technology—initial clinical results. J Am Coll Cardiol 2004;44:1230–7.
12. Raff GL, Gallagher MJ, O'Neill WW, et al. Diagnostic accuracy of noninvasive coronary angiography using 64-slice spiral computed tomography. J Am Coll Cardiol 2005;46:552–7.
13. Leber AW, Knez A, von Ziegler F, et al. Quantification of obstructive and nonobstructive coronary lesions by 64-slice computed tomography: a comparative study with quantitative coronary angiography and intravascular ultrasound. J Am Coll Cardiol 2005;46:147–54.
14. Mollet NR, Cademartiri F, van Mieghan CA, et al. High-resolution spiral computed tomography coronary angiography in patients referred for diagnostic conventional coronary angiography. Circulation 2005;112:2318–23.
15. Rius T, Goyenechea M, Poon M. Combined cardiac congenital anomalies assessed by multislice spiral computed tomography. Eur Heart J 2006;27(6):637.

16. Watkins MW, Hesse B, Green CE, et al. Detection of coronary artery stenosis using 40-channel computed tomography with multisegment reconstruction. Am J Cardiol 2007;99:175–81.
17. Miller JM, Rochitte CE, Dewey M, et al. Diagnostic performance of coronary angiography by 64-row CT. N Engl J Med 2008;359(22):2324–36.
18. Budoff MJ, Dowe D, Jollis JG, et al. Diagnostic performance of 64-multidetector row coronary computed tomographic angiography for evaluation of coronary artery stenosis in individuals without known coronary artery disease: results from the prospective multicenter ACCURACY (Assessment by Coronary Computed Tomographic Angiography of Individuals Undergoing Invasive Coronary Angiography) trial. J Am Coll Cardiol 2008;52(21):1724–32.
19. Nissen SE, Grinses CL, Gurley JC, et al. Application of a new phased-away ultrasound imaging catheter in the assessment of vascular dimensions: in vivo comparison to cine angiography. Circulation 1980; 81:660–6.
20. Vince D, Dixon K, Cothern R, et al. Comparison of texture analysis methods for the characterization of coronary plaques in intravascular ultrasound images. Comput Med Imaging Graph 2000;24(4): 221–9.
21. Kostamaa H, Donoran J, Kasaoka E, et al. Calcified plaque cross-sectional area in human arteries: correlation between intravascular ultrasound and undercalcified histology. Am Heart J 1999;3:482–8.
22. Kopp A, Schoroeder S, Baumbach A, et al. Noninvasive characterization lesion morphology and composition by multislice: just results in comparison with intracoronary ultrasound. Eur Radiol 2001;11(9): 1607–11.
23. Tobis JM, Mallery JA, Gessert J, et al. Intravascular ultrasound cross-sectional arterial imaging before and after balloon angioplasty in vitro. Circulation 1989;70:873–82.
24. Schoenhagen P, Tuzcu EM, Stillman AE, et al. Non-invasive assessment of plaque morphology and remodeling in mildly stenotic coronary segments: comparison of 16-slice computed tomography and intravascular ultrasound. Coron Artery Dis 2003;14:459–62.
25. Achenbach S, Moselewski F, Ropers D, et al. Detection of calcified and noncalcified coronary atherosclerotic plaque by contrast-enhanced, submillimeter multidetector spiral computed tomography. A segment-based comparison with intravascular ultrasound. Circulation 2004;109:14–7.
26. Saad EB, Rossillo A, Saad CP, et al. Pulmonary vein stenosis after radiofrequency ablation of atrial fibrillation: functional characterization, evolution, and influence of the ablation strategy. Circulation 2003; 108:3102–7.
27. Restrepo CS, Largoza A, Lemos DF, et al. CT and MR imaging findings of malignant cardiac tumors. Curr Probl Diagn Radiol 2005;34(1):1–11.
28. Hachamovitch R, Hayes SW, Friedman JD, et al. Identification of a threshold of inducible ischemia associated with a short-term survival benefit with revascularization compared to medical therapy in patients with no prior cad undergoing stress myocardial perfusion SPECT. Circulation 2003;107: 2899–906.
29. Flohr TG, McCollough CH, Bruder H, et al. First performance evaluation of a dual-source CT (DSCT)system. Eur Radiol 2006;16:256–68.
30. Weustink AC, Meijboom WB, Mollet NR, et al. Reliable high-speed coronary computed tomography in symptomatic patients. J Am Coll Cardiol 2007; 50(8):786–94.
31. Endo M, Mori S, Tsunoo T, et al. Development and performance evaluation of the first model of 4D CT-scanner. IEEE Trans Nucl Sci 2003;50:1667–71.
32. Mori S, Nishizawa K, Kondo C, et al. Effective doses in subjects undergoing computed tomography cardiac imaging with the 256-multislice CT scanner. Eur J Radiol 2008;65(3):442–8.
33. Shuman WP, Branch KR, May JM, et al. Prospective versus retrospective ECG gating for 64-detector CT of the coronary arteries: comparison of image quality and patient radiation dose. Radiology 2008; 248:431–7.

# Diagnostic Accuracy of CT Coronary Angiography

Divya Kapoor, MD[a], Randall C. Thompson, MD[a,b,c,*]

**KEYWORDS**

- Coronary CT angiography • Accuracy
- Angiographic correlation • Correlation with Stress Test
- Maximizing accuracy

Coronary artery disease (CAD) remains a leading cause of mortality and morbidity in the United States and most Western countries, and cardiac imaging plays an important role in the diagnosis and management of patients who have CAD. Although it is clear that coronary computed tomography angiography (CTA) sometimes can provide images of superb diagnostic quality, and the agreement with invasive coronary angiogram is sometimes exquisite (see **Fig. 1**), it also is obvious that the image quality of coronary CTA sometimes can be challenging. CTA is, of course, a new diagnostic test compared with other established modalities. There now is a rich and rapidly growing literature on the diagnostic utility of coronary CTA and its performance relative to other modalities such as stress testing and invasive coronary angiography. Elsewhere in this issue, Garcia reviews the important concerns relative to adopting a new diagnostic modality for clinical practice. This article reviews the key literature regarding the accuracy and limitations of coronary CTA, a crucial feature to consider in determining the proper role of this diagnostic tool.

## COMPARISON OF CORONARY CT ANGIOGRAPHY AND OTHER DIAGNOSTIC MODALITIES

### *Cardiac Catheterization*

Since the introduction of 16-slice CT instrumentation, numerous publications have compared the results of coronary CTA and those of invasive coronary angiography. Although the diagnostic quality of CT angiograms, which have superb image quality, is excellent, even recent publications that study the latest techniques show that the diagnostic accuracy is imperfect in comparison with the reference standard of invasive coronary angiography. **Table 1** lists recent meta-analyses of comparisons of CTA and invasive coronary angiography. Most of the patients studied were referred for invasive cardiac catheterization because of clinical indications and underwent both procedures. Earlier studies of 16-slice coronary CTA showed wide variability in sensitivity (30%–95%) and some variability in specificity (86%–98%).[4,6–16] Despite good overall diagnostic accuracy, several studies were limited because un-interpretable segments were excluded from the analysis.

One multicenter study, by Garcia and colleagues,[17] evaluated the accuracy of 16-slice coronary CTA and its routine use in diagnosing CAD. Using rigorous methodology, this study had to exclude 29% segments as un-evaluable. In the analysis these segments were "censored as positive"; sensitivity, specificity, negative predictive value, and positive predictive values were 89%, 65%, 99%, 13%, respectively. This study, which used a central core laboratory for interpretation, demonstrated a lower specificity with a higher rate of false positives than reported

[a] Division of Cardiovascular Diseases, University of Missouri Kansas City, Mid America Heart Institute, 4330 Wornall Road, Kansas City, MO 64111, USA
[b] University of Missouri Kansas City, Mid America Heart Institute, 4401 Wornall Road, Kansas City, MO 64111, USA
[c] Cardiovascular Consultants, PA, Kansas City, 4330 Wornall Road, Kansas City, MO 64111, USA
* Corresponding author.
*E-mail address:* rthompson@cc-pc.com (R.C. Thompson).

Cardiol Clin 27 (2009) 563–571
doi:10.1016/j.ccl.2009.06.011

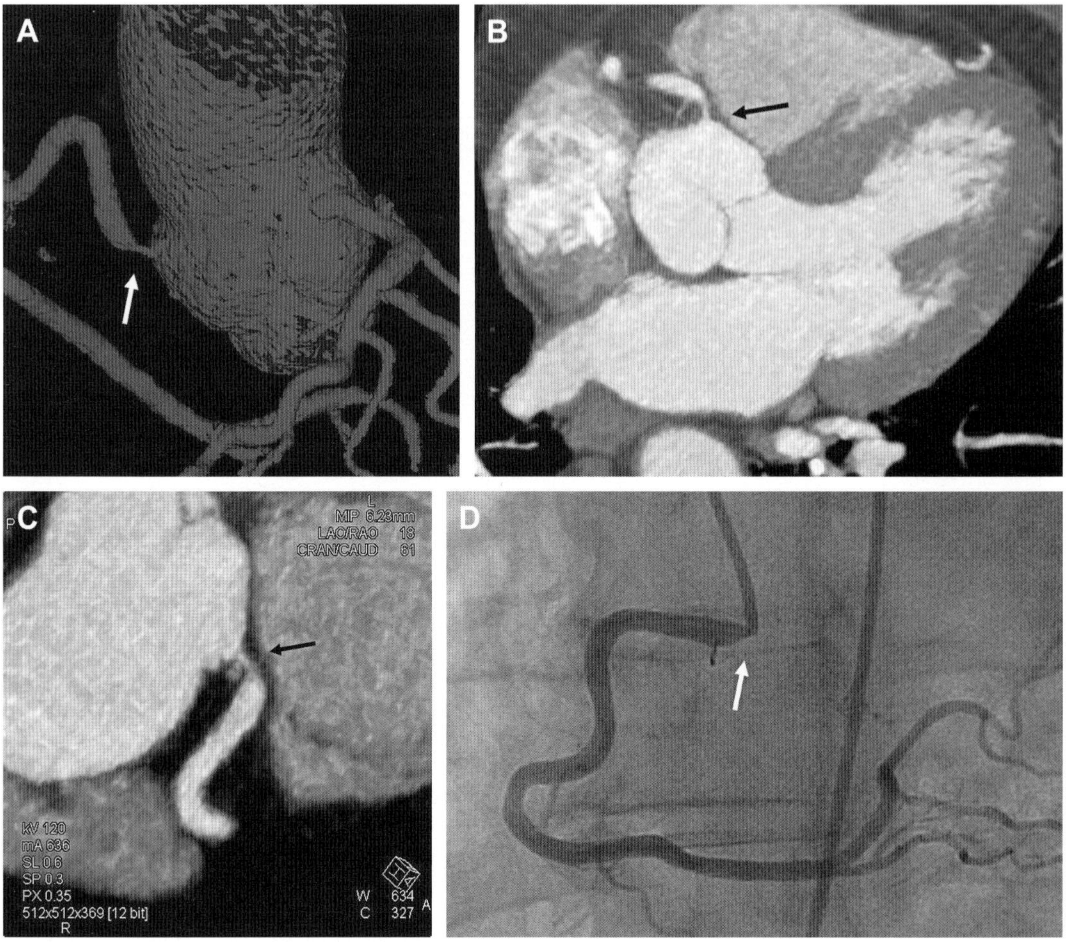


**Fig. 1.** Volume-rendered CTA (*A*) and maximum intensity projection (*B* and *C*) coronary CTA along with invasive coronary angiogram (*D*) in a patient who has a high-grade ostial right coronary artery stenosis (*arrows* in *A–D*).

in previous analyses that had excluded un-evaluable segments. It should be noted, however, that the negative predictive value of 16-slice coronary CTA is excellent, both in the single-center publications and in the multicenter trial mentioned previously. Thus, a coronary CTA of good diagnostic quality that shows no coronary stenosis can be said to exclude significant CAD.

With 40- and 64-slice coronary CTA, more of the chest is covered with each spin of the gantry, the breath hold is shorter, and there are fewer uninterpretable segments than with 16-slice coronary CTA. Also, concomitant improvements in scanner designs by some manufacturers have improved the spatial and temporal resolution with new iterations of 64-slice scanners. As **Table 1** shows, the overall accuracy is substantially better with 40- or 64-slice coronary CTA than in previous reports with 16-slice scanners.

Recent individual studies of 64-slice coronary CTA, including a multicenter investigation by Miller and colleagues,[18] demonstrate rather high sensitivity, specificity, negative predictive accuracy, and positive predictive values (85%, 90%, 83%, and 91%, respectively) when compared with invasive angiography. The study by Miller and colleagues did exclude patients who had a calcium score higher than 600 and segments smaller than 1.5 mm in diameter, because they were considered un-evaluable. Similarly, in another study by Raff and colleagues,[19] 83% of segments were quantifiable, and the sensitivity, specificity, negative predictive value, and positive predictive value per segment were 95%, 86%, 98%, and 66%, respectively, when compared with invasive coronary angiography. The per-patient–based analysis revealed better overall accuracy with sensitivity, specificity, positive predictive value, and negative predictive values of 90%, 95%, 93%, and 93%, respectively. Similarly in another study by Mollet and colleagues,[20] the patient-based analysis revealed 100% sensitivity and 100% negative

**Table 1**
**Systematic reviews: studies of patient-based analysis using 64-slice coronary CTA**

| Study | Sensitivity (%) | Specificity (%) | PPV (%) | NPV (%) | Year | N |
|---|---|---|---|---|---|---|
| Stein et al.[1] | 98 | 88 | 93 | 96 | 2008 | 2045 |
| Mowatt et al.[2] | 99 | 89 | 93[b] | 100[b] | 2008 | 1286 |
| Abdulla et al.[3] | 98 | 91 | 94 | 97 | 2007 | 875 |
| Gopalalkrishnan et al.[4,a] | 96 | 91 | 93 | 96 | 2008 | 596 |
| Sun et al.[5] | 97 | 88 | 94 | 95 | 2008 | 1027 |

*Abbreviations:* NPV, negative predictive value; PPV, positive predictive value.
[a] This analysis included one study with 40-slice MDCT.
[b] PPV and NPV were reported as median values.

predictive value. These findings are consistent with the results of other investigators shown in a systematic review of 64-slice CTA in **Tables 1** and **2**.

A multicenter study by Budoff and colleagues[21] included consecutive patients undergoing 64-slice CTA and all available coronary segments. The analysis showed sensitivity and specificity of 95% and 83%, respectively, and negative and positive predictive values of 99% and 44%, respectively. Thus, coronary CTA has clear diagnostic utility. The very high negative predictive value is especially valuable in ruling out coronary artery disease in patients who have a low to intermediate pretest likelihood of CAD.

In the studies included in **Tables 1** and **2**, a reduction of 50% in the diameter of the coronary artery lumen generally was considered significant, but some studies evaluated a stenosis of 70% or more as a cutoff. **Table 1** lists data from patient-based analyses, and **Table 2** lists data from coronary-based analyses. Although earlier publications with limited numbers of patients calculated accuracy by segment or artery, accuracy based on patient analysis is more clinically relevant. For example, a coronary CT angiogram in which 16 of 17 segments correlate well with angiography but which missed an important coronary stenosis in the other segment would have a high per-segment accuracy but appropriately would be considered inaccurate in that patient. As the tables show, CTA has a lower positive predictive value with segment-based analysis than with patient-based analysis, but the negative predictive values are similar. These data suggest that coronary CTA cannot supplant coronary angiography in determining which vessels have critical coronary stenosis and need revascularization. Coronary CTA, however, seems to be extremely reliable in ruling out critical coronary artery disease and excluding patients who do not require further evaluation by invasive angiography. In fact, this strong negative predictive accuracy is cited as the reason for preferentially performing coronary CTA in patients who have chest pain and a low to intermediate pretest likelihood of coronary stenosis.[22]

### *Stress Testing*

Invasive coronary angiography and coronary CTA are anatomic techniques; that is, they display the anatomic changes of coronary disease. In contrast, other diagnostic tests for CAD, such as myocardial perfusion imaging and stress echocardiography, are physiologic tests and estimate the interruption of myocardial nutrient flow caused by coronary atherosclerotic disease. A number of reports have compared the performance of measures of stenoses by coronary CTA with measures of ischemia by myocardial perfusion imaging. **Table 3** lists some of these data. When compared with ischemia detected by myocardial perfusion imaging, coronary CTA is sensitive and has a high negative predictive value but has a fairly low specificity. Only about half the patients who had CTA segments that appeared to have significant stenoses had significant ischemia on myocardial perfusion imaging.[23–26] Coronary CTA is superior to other noninvasive cardiac imaging studies in detecting early/subclinical CAD, but because a fair number of stenoses that appear to be significant by CTA do not correlate with ischemic defects on stress testing, both types of tests maybe necessary in some patients, particularly when anatomic coronary disease is established by CTA but symptoms are mild or atypical.

## ACCURACY OF CORONARY CT ANGIOGRAPHY IN SPECIAL PATIENT POPULATIONS

### *Accuracy in In-stent Restenosis*

Coronary CTA offers a noninvasive method to evaluate stent patency, a clinically relevant issue in the management of many patients who have

**Table 2**
**Systematic reviews: studies of segment-based analysis using 64-slice coronary CTA**

| Study | Sensitivity (%) | Specificity (%) | PPV (%) | NPV (%) | Year | Segments | Un-Evaluable Segments |
|---|---|---|---|---|---|---|---|
| Stein et al.[1] | 90[a] | 96[a] | 73[a] | 99[a] | 2008 | 32,046 | 7.8% |
| Mowatt et al.[2] | 90[a] | 97[a] | 76[a,c] | 99[a,c] | 2008 | 14,199 | 8% |
| Abdulla et al.[3] | 86[a] | 96[a] | 83[a] | 97[a] | 2007 | 17,695 | 4% |
| Gopalakrishnanet al.[4,d] | 91[a] | 96[a] | 78[a] | 98[a] | 2008 | Not all specified | 4%, but not all specified |
| Sun et al.[5] | 92[b]/90[a] | 92[b]/96[a] | 78[b]/75[a] | 98[b]/98[a] | 2008 | Not all specified | Not all specified |

*Abbreviations:* NPV, negative predictive value; PPV, positive predictive value.
[a] Segment-based analysis.
[b] Vessel-based analysis.
[c] PPV and NPV were reported as median values.
[d] This analysis included one study with 40-slice MDCT.

**Table 3**
**Comparison of myocardial perfusion images (MPI) with coronary CTA**

| Study | Sensitivity (%) | Specificity (%) | PPV (%) | NPV (%) | Year | N | Type of MPI |
|---|---|---|---|---|---|---|---|
| Gaemperli et al.[23,c] | 95[a]/95[b] | 53[a]/75[b] | 58[a]/72[b] | 94[a]/96[b] | 2008 | 78 | SPECT |
| Di Carli et al.[24,d] | 68[a]/61[b] | 78[a]/87[b] | 44[a]/26[b] | 91[a]/97[b] | 2007 | 110 | PET-CT |
| Haramati et al.[25,e] | 73[a] | 80[a] | 55[a] | 90[a] | 2008 | 61 | SPECT |
| Nicol et al.[26,c] | 100[a] | 84[a] | 50[a] | 100[a] | 2008 | 52 | SPECT |

*Abbreviations:* NPV, negative predictive value; PET, positron emission tomography; PPV, positive predictive value; SPECT, single photon emission computed tomography.
[a] Patient-based analysis.
[b] Vessel-based analysis.
[c] Stenosis $\geq$ 50% was considered significant.
[d] Stenosis between 50% and 70% was used for this analysis.
[e] Stenosis $\geq$ 70% was considered significant for this analysis.

undergone percutaneous revascularization. Stent struts cause beam hardening artifact, however, and these segments are not always evaluable by CTA. For larger stents, there is an emerging consensus that CTA is clinically useful. One study compared CTA with invasive angiography and intravascular ultrasound during cardiac catheterization to evaluate left main stent patency.[27] This study showed good correlation of CTA with both invasive coronary angiogram (ICA) and intravascular ultrasound, and the overall accuracy was 93%. The accuracy of CTA for determining patency of left main stents was 98%, but it was significantly lower for bifurcation stents (83%) with more false-positive results.[27] The negative predictive accuracy for CTA was 100% in this study. Although in the United States bypass surgery still is usually considered the standard of care for most patients who have left main stenosis, stenting of the left main coronary artery is performed frequently, especially in other countries. In the past, follow-up myocardial perfusion imaging was not considered accurate enough to detect restenosis in these patients, and routine follow-up coronary angiography has been the custom in many practices. Based on the report by Van Mieghem and colleagues,[27] coronary CTA would seem to be a reasonable alternative to coronary angiography in this subgroup of patients.

Studies on the accuracy of CTA to determine in-stent restenosis in locations other than the left main artery (where the stents tend to be smaller in diameter and the arteries more prone to motion) have been mixed. For example, in one study by Rixe and colleagues,[28] CTA for in-stent restenosis had a sensitivity of 50% and specificity of 57%. When the stent segments were further stratified as evaluable or un-evaluable, however, the sensitivity and specificity increased significantly, to 86% and 98%, respectively, in the evaluable cases.[28] In a systematic review of this subject by Mowatt and colleagues,[2] the number of un-evaluable stented segments was as high as 21% in some studies, and the average sensitivity and specificity were 89% and 94%, respectively. Another recent meta-analysis by Vanhoenacker and colleagues[29] showed moderate sensitivity (82%) and good specificity (91%), although there was heterogeneity in the types of studies that were pooled, and the categorization of stents as un-evaluable was influenced by the type of CT scanner used, stent diameter, strut thickness, and edge-enhancing kernels. In another study by Cademartiri and colleagues,[30] which compared coronary CTA with invasive coronary angiography for in-stent restenosis, the negative predictive value of CTA for stents with diameter of 2.5 mm or larger was 99% , but 7% of stented segments were un-evaluable because of poor image quality.

As mentioned earlier, stents can cause blooming and beam-hardening artifacts on CTA images. There is an emerging consensus that CTA can be useful for the determination of stenosis in most stents larger than 3 mm and in some as small as 2.5 mm in diameter. The accuracy of CTA in detecting in-stent restenosis depends on the both the complexity of the stented lesion and type of stent. These features should be considered when trying to exclude coronary artery stenosis using this modality.

## *Accuracy in Bypass Grafts*

Although there are numerous studies evaluating the sensitivity and specificity of coronary CTA in native vessels and segments, there are only a few reports of the use of CTA in the evaluation of bypass grafts. In a study by Ropers and colleagues,[31] CTA images of 138 grafts, native vessels, and anastomotic sites were compared with invasive coronary angiograms. The grafts included both venous and arterial bypass conduits. All the grafts were evaluable by coronary CTA, with sensitivity, specificity, and positive and negative predictive values of 100%, 94%, 92%, and 100%, respectively, indicating very high accuracy. **Table 4** lists the results of four systematic reviews that evaluated the accuracy of CTA when compared with invasive angiography for coronary bypass grafts.

Coronary CTA has a high level of accuracy in the detecting clinically significant CAD in bypass grafts. Although metallic clips sometimes can obscure portions of a bypass graft body, they rarely interfere with the detection of stenoses. In these patients, however, distal coronary anastomotic sites and distal native coronary segments sometimes are small and obscured by dense calcification. Thus, in most cases, the CTA has limited clinical utility in evaluating graft patency and graft stenosis.

### *Coronary CT Angiography and Coronary Anomalies*

Coronary anomalies can be demonstrated by conventional invasive angiography, but the two-dimensional depiction of the course of these complex three-dimensional structures is inherently limited. Because of the three-dimensional display and the ability to image surrounding anatomic structures such as the ascending aorta and pulmonary artery, coronary CTA can be a very valuable tool both in diagnosing coronary anomalies and in providing detailed information about them.

In a case series by Kacmaz and colleagues,[32] CTA was compared with traditional coronary angiography in diagnosing coronary anomalies. CTA had 100% sensitivity and provided important detailed anatomic information. Another case series by Ten Kate and colleagues[33] evaluated 1000 patients for the diagnoses of anomalous coronary artery from opposite sinus (ACAOS) and coronary arterial fistulae. In this series, all five patients who had right ACAOS had previously undergone invasive angiography with unsuccessful detection of the right coronary artery, which was visualized by CTA.

CTA can be an especially helpful tool in depicting another form of coronary abnormality, myocardial bridging. The three-dimensional display of CTA easily demonstrates the course of the coronary artery when it passes through the myocardium. In one study of myocardial bridging by Leschka and colleagues,[34] all patients underwent both conventional angiograms and CTA. In this study, only 46% of patients who had a bridge identified by CTA were diagnosed by invasive angiography. Lower depth, smaller length, and lower systolic compression of the tunneled segment of the coronary correlated with missed diagnosis on the conventional angiogram.

## LIMITATIONS OF CORONARY CT ANGIOGRAPHY AND METHODS FOR MAXIMIZING ACCURACY

Coronary CTA, although a precise technique, does have several limitations that interfere with its accuracy. These limitations include vascular calcification, limited temporal and spatial resolution, and motion artifacts.

Calcium in the epicardial coronaries is a very sensitive indicator of CAD. Unfortunately, dense calcified plaques create blooming artifact on CT images that can decrease the specificity of coronary CTA to detect coronary stenoses. Although a number of experts believe that coronary CTAs

**Table 4**
**Accuracy of CTA in bypass grafts**

| Study | Sensitivity of Stenosis in Patent Grafts (%) | Specificity of Stenosis in Patent Grafts (%) | PPV (%) | NPV (%) | Year | Un-Evaluable Graft Segments |
|---|---|---|---|---|---|---|
| Stein et al.[1] | 98 | 97 | 92 | 99 | 2008 | At least 7%; not all specified |
| Abdulla et al.[3] | 99 | 96 | 92 | 99 | 2007 | 0 |
| Gopalakrishnan et al.[4,a] | 97 | 97 | 87 | 97 | 2008 | 7%, but not all studies specified |
| Mowatt et al.[2] | 99 | 96 | 93[b] | 99[b] | 2008 | 0 |

*Abbreviations:* NPV, negative predictive value; PPV, positive predictive value.
[a] This analysis included 1 study with 40-slice MDCT.
[b] PPV and NPV in this study were reported at median values.

have diagnostic value in almost all patients who have high calcium scores, many studies have excluded vessels or patients if the calcium score is above a certain Agaston number. For example, Miller and colleagues[18] proposed a cutoff of 600 Agatston units and suggested that the test would be best performed only in patients with scores below this number. Also, some randomized trials such as the one by Budoff and colleagues[21] evaluated the results in patients whose Agatston scores were greater than 400. In this multicenter prospective trial (Assessment by Coronary Computed Tomographic Angiography of Individuals Undergoing Invasive Coronary Angiograph, ACCURACY) none of the patients was excluded from the study based on calcium score. This investigation found that the diagnosis of obstructive CAD in patients who had an Agaston score of 400 or less had a specificity of 86.3%, but when patients who had an Agaston score higher than 400 were included, the specificity fell to 52.6%.[21] Calcified plaques cause blooming effects (an enlarged appearance), as do stents, making a stenosis appear more severe than it is in reality.

Although coronary CTA technology has achieved a high level of accuracy in detecting patients who have obstructive coronary artery disease, it lacks sufficient accuracy to identify all stenotic lesions in a given patient; therefore it cannot yet be used routinely to guide therapy in patients who have CAD. As discussed earlier, some of this limitation is related to obscuring coronary calcium, and diagnostic quality often is inadequate in heavily calcified coronary segments. Calcium is much less of a confounder for invasive angiography because the spatial resolution is superior and the concentration of iodinated contrast is higher in the coronary arteries than achieved with CTA.

Temporal resolution also is somewhat suboptimal with coronary CTA. Temporal resolution is determined primarily by the speed of the rotating X-ray gantry, which is limited by the weight of the gantry and the laws of physics. Beta-blockers are used routinely to slow the heart rate, but residual motion of the coronary arteries in the CT image sometimes causes blurred coronary segments, and this motion is a source of inaccuracy. Elsewhere in this issue, Halliburton discusses some of the recent technological advances in multidetector cardiac CT, including those that help mitigate the problem of temporal resolution. Patient motion and respiratory movement also can cause a loss of accuracy with CTA, and careful attention to patient preparation and instructions is important in minimizing these problems.

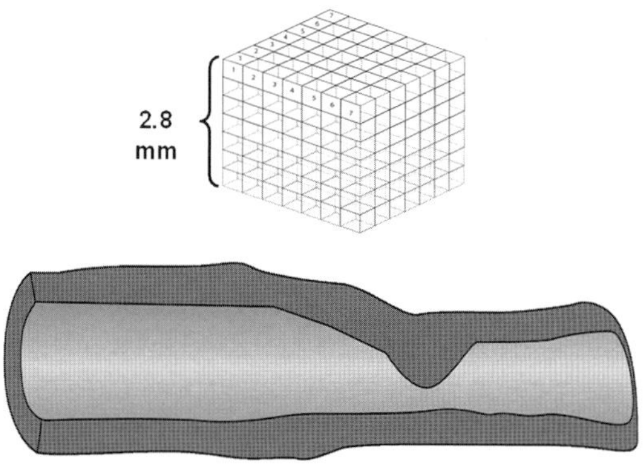


**Fig. 2.** Limitation of spatial resolution of coronary CTA.

Coronary CTA does have an important advantage over invasive angiography in that it is an inherently three-dimensional technique. In certain cases, the two-dimensional display of a coronary angiogram is a significant limitation, as in determining the severity of ostial left main stenosis, visualizing severely overlapping vessels, determining the course of an occluded artery, or determining the course of coronary artery anomalies. In these cases, the three-dimensional display of coronary CTA may make it superior to invasive coronary angiography despite the lower resolution. These patients sometimes are referred for CTA after an invasive angiogram.

The maximum spatial resolution of multidetector CT is 0.4 to 0.8 mm. This resolution is determined in large part by the size of the picture elements of the CT detector. As discussed earlier, smaller coronary segments frequently are un-evaluable with CTA. Also, coronary CTA frequently is unable to distinguish moderate stenoses, which presumably are not flow limiting (eg, a reduction in diameter of 40%), from moderately severe or severe stenoses, which presumably are flow limiting (ie, a reduction in diameter of70%). **Fig. 2** illustrates this limitation of spatial resolution and how it affects discrimination of stenosis severity in the intermediate range. For a coronary segment that is 2.8 mm in diameter, there may be a difference of only one to four picture elements between a stenosis of 30% to 40% and one that has a reduction in diameter of 70% to 80% (**Fig. 2**).

## SUMMARY

Coronary CTA, although having a high degree of accuracy, sometimes is limited by suboptimal image quality. Heavy coronary calcifications, motion artifact, and limitations of temporal and spatial resolution occasionally result in images that do not correlate well with invasive coronary angiographic measures of the severity of CAD. When image quality is excellent, however, coronary CTA is very reliable, especially in ruling out obstructive CAD in patients who have low to intermediate pretest likelihood of disease. This modality also has reasonable accuracy and an emerging clinical role in determining the patency of moderate to large-sized coronary stents, especially stents in the left main position, and is accurate in determining the patency of coronary bypass grafts. Coronary CTA, because it is inherently three-dimensional, also has important advantages over other modalities, including invasive angiography. It is a preferred modality for evaluating coronary and other cardiac anomalies and has potential advantages in patients who have ostial arterial stenoses. In its current state, CTA cannot replace invasive coronary angiography, especially for guiding decisions of revascularization, but it is a valuable tool in a number of patient groups.

## REFERENCES


1. Stein PD, Yaekoub AY, Matta F, et al. 64-slice CT for diagnosis of coronary artery disease: a systematic review. Am J Med 2008;121(8):715–25.
2. Mowatt G, Cook JA, Hillis GS, et al. 64-slice computed tomography angiography in the diagnosis and assessment of coronary artery disease: systematic review and meta-analysis. Heart 2008; 94(11):1386–93.
3. Abdulla J, Abildstrom SZ, Gotzsche O, et al. 64-multislice detector computed tomography coronary angiography as potential alternative to conventional coronary angiography: a systematic review and meta-analysis. Eur Heart J 2007;28(24):3042–50.
4. Gopalakrishnan P, Wilson GT, Tak T. Accuracy of multislice computed tomography coronary angiography: a pooled estimate. Cardiol Rev 2008;16(4): 189–96.
5. Sun Z, Lin C, Davidson R, et al. Diagnostic value of 64-slice CT angiography in coronary artery disease: a systematic review. Eur J Radiol 2008;67(1):78–84.
6. d'Othee B, Janne U, Siebert R, et al. A systematic review on diagnostic accuracy of CT-based detection of significant coronary artery disease. Eur J Radiol 2008;65(3):449–61.
7. Ropers D, Baum U, Pohle K, et al. Detection of coronary artery stenoses with thin-slice multi-detector row spiral computed tomography and multiplanar reconstruction. Circulation 2003;107(5):664–6.
8. Hoffmann MH, Shi H, Schmitz BL, et al. Noninvasive coronary angiography with multislice computed tomography. JAMA 2005;293(20):2471–8.
9. Achenbach S, Ropers D, Pohle FK, et al. Detection of coronary artery stenoses using multi-detector CT with 16 × 0.75 collimation and 375 ms rotation. Eur Heart J 2005;26(19):1978–86.
10. Mollet NR, Cademartiri F, Krestin GP, et al. Improved diagnostic accuracy with 16-row multi-slice computed tomography coronary angiography. J Am Coll Cardiol 2005;45(1):128–32.
11. Kuettner A, Beck T, Drosch T, et al. Image quality and diagnostic accuracy of non-invasive coronary imaging with 16 detector slice spiral computed tomography with 188 ms temporal resolution. Heart 2005;91(7):938–41.
12. Nieman K, Cademartiri F, Lemos PA, et al. Reliable noninvasive coronary angiography with fast submillimeter multislice spiral computed tomography. Circulation 2002;106(16):2051–4.
13. Kuettner A, Beck T, Drosch T, et al. Diagnostic accuracy of noninvasive coronary imaging using 16-detector slice spiral computed tomography with 188 ms temporal resolution. J Am Coll Cardiol 2005;45(1):123–7.
14. Kaiser C, Bremerich J, Haller S, et al. Limited diagnostic yield of non-invasive coronary angiography by 16-slice multi-detector spiral computed tomography in routine patients referred for evaluation of coronary artery disease. Eur Heart J 2005;26(19): 1987–92.
15. Dewey M, Laule M, Krug L, et al. Multisegment and halfscan reconstruction of 16-slice computed tomography for detection of coronary artery stenoses. Invest Radiol 2004;39(4):223–9.
16. Kuettner A, Trabold T, Schroeder S, et al. Noninvasive detection of coronary lesions using 16-detector multislice spiral computed tomography technology: initial clinical results. J Am Coll Cardiol 2004;44(6): 1230–7.
17. Garcia MJ, Lessick J, Hoffmann MH. Accuracy of 16-row multidetector computed tomography for the assessment of coronary artery stenosis. JAMA 2006;296(4):403–11.
18. Miller JM, Rochitte CE, Dewey M, et al. Diagnostic performance of coronary angiography by 64-row CT. N Engl J Med 2008;359(22):2324–36.
19. Raff GL, Gallagher MJ, O'Neill WW, et al. Diagnostic accuracy of noninvasive coronary angiography using 64-slice spiral computed tomography. J Am Coll Cardiol 2005;46(3):552–7.
20. Mollet NR, Cademartiri F, Van Mieghem CA, et al. High-resolution spiral computed tomography coronary angiography in patients referred for diagnostic conventional coronary angiography. Circulation 2005;112(15):2318–23.
21. Budoff MJ, Dowe D, Jollis JG, et al. Diagnostic performance of 64-multidetector row coronary computed tomographic angiography for evaluation of coronary artery stenosis in individuals without known coronary artery disease: results from the prospective multicenter ACCURACY (Assessment by Coronary

Computed Tomographic Angiography of Individuals Undergoing Invasive Coronary Angiography) trial. J Am Coll Cardiol 2008;52(21):1724–32.
22. Thompson RC, Thomas GS, Yasuda T, et al. Potential indications for coronary angiography by computed tomography. Am Heart Hosp J 2005; 3(3):161–6, 174.
23. Gaemperli O, Schepis T, Valenta I, et al. Functionally relevant coronary artery disease: comparison of 64-section CT angiography with myocardial perfusion SPECT. Radiology 2008;248(2):414–23.
24. Di Carli MF, Dorbala S, Curillova Z, et al. Relationship between CT coronary angiography and stress perfusion imaging in patients with suspected ischemic heart disease assessed by integrated PET-CT imaging. J Nucl Cardiol 2007;14(6): 799–809.
25. Haramati LB, Levsky JM, Jain VR, et al. CT angiography for evaluation of coronary artery disease in inner-city outpatients: an initial prospective comparison with stress myocardial perfusion imaging. Int J Cardiovasc Imaging 2009;25(3):303–13.
26. Nicol ED, Stirrup J, Reyes E, et al. Sixty-four-slice computed tomography coronary angiography compared with myocardial perfusion scintigraphy for the diagnosis of functionally significant coronary stenoses in patients with a low to intermediate likelihood of coronary artery disease. J Nucl Cardiol 2008;15(3):311–8.
27. Van Mieghem CA, Cademartiri F, Mollet NR, et al. Multislice spiral computed tomography for the evaluation of stent patency after left main coronary artery stenting: a comparison with conventional coronary angiography and intravascular ultrasound. Circulation 2006;114(7):645–53.
28. Rixe J, Achenbach S, Ropers D, et al. Assessment of coronary artery stent restenosis by 64-slice multidetector computed tomography. Eur Heart J 2006; 27(21):2567–72.
29. Vanhoenacker PK, Decramer I, Bladt O, et al. Multidetector computed tomography angiography for assessment of in-stent restenosis: meta-analysis of diagnostic performance. BMC Med Imaging 2008; 8:14.
30. Cademartiri F, Schuijf JD, Pugliese F, et al. Usefulness of 64-slice multislice computed tomography coronary angiography to assess in-stent restenosis. J Am Coll Cardiol 2007;49(22):2204–10.
31. Ropers D, Pohle FK, Kuettner A, et al. Diagnostic accuracy of noninvasive coronary angiography in patients after bypass surgery using 64-slice spiral computed tomography with 330-ms gantry rotation. Circulation 2006;114(22):2334–41.
32. Kacmaz F, Ozbulbul NI, Alyan O, et al. Imaging of coronary artery anomalies: the role of multidetector computed tomography. Coron Artery Dis 2008; 19(3):203–9.
33. Ten Kate GJ, Weustink AC, de Feyter PJ. Coronary artery anomalies detected by MSCT-coronary angiography in the adult. Neth Heart J 2008;16(11): 369–75.
34. Leschka S, Koepfli P, Husmann L, et al. Myocardial bridging: depiction rate and morphology at CT coronary angiography—comparison with conventional coronary angiography. Radiology 2008;246(3): 754–62.

# The Prognostic Value of Cardiac Computed Tomographic Angiography

Fay Y. Lin, MD, MSc, Suzanne E. Zentko, MD, James K. Min, MD*

**KEYWORDS**

- Cardiac computed tomographic angiography
- Prognosis • Risk stratification • Predictive value

Precise risk stratification by cardiac computed tomographic angiography (CCTA) necessitates accurate visualization and diagnosis of coronary artery atherosclerosis.[1–3] Prior studies have focused upon the diagnostic performance of CCTA for the detection and exclusion of obstructive coronary artery stenosis, and more than 50 studies have been published in this regard. Recently, multiple prospective multicenter trials have demonstrated excellent diagnostic characteristics of 64-detector row CCTA in comparison to invasive coronary angiography (ICA) in appropriate patients.[1,4,5] The ACCURACY trial (Assessment by Coronary Computed Tomographic Angiography of Individuals Undergoing Invasive Coronary Angiography), a 15-center United States-based multicenter study examining 230 patients undergoing CCTA before elective ICA observed sensitivity, specificity, and positive (PPV) and negative predictive values (NPV) of CCTA to detect a greater than or equal to 50% or greater than or equal to 70% stenosis of 95%, 83%, 64%, and 99%, respectively, and 94% 83%, 48%, and 99% respectively. The high sensitivity and NPV of CCTA compares favorably to more traditionally employed functional imaging modalities, such as exercise echocardiography and myocardial perfusion-gated single-photon emission computed tomography (SPECT) imaging (MPS) for detection and exclusion of significant intraluminal stenosis.[2]

These CCTA measures of intraluminal stenosis severity have been examined for their relation to functional imaging findings with known prognostic significance. Among 169 low-to-intermediate risk patients who underwent both exercise treadmill testing and CCTA, the presence of obstructive ($\geq$70%) stenosis was associated with both ST segment depression [adjusted odds ratio (OR) 3.38 (1.32, 8.64), $P$ = .001] and elevated risk Duke treadmill scores [adjusted OR 4.67 (1.97, 11.03), $P$<.001], with a graded relationship between the burden of coronary artery disease by a modified Duke coronary artery jeopardy score and the exercise time, as well as the likelihood of ST segment depression ($P$<.05 for both).[6] Among 163 low-to-intermediate risk patients who underwent both MPS and CCTA, the global burden of coronary artery plaque as measured by a modified Duke coronary artery jeopardy score was independently associated with severely abnormal MPS scans [OR 2.25 (1.12–4.41), $P$ = .02 for the highest risk group compared with those without disease].[7] It is notable that CCTA measures beyond intraluminal stenosis severity—including extraluminal plaque composition—were also associated with the same surrogate endpoints of elevated risk, with greater numbers of "mixed" plaques (that is, admixtures of calcified and noncalcified plaques) observed in individuals with higher likelihoods of ST segment depression, higher-risk Duke

Department of Medicine, Division of Cardiology, Weill Medical College of Cornell University, New York Presbyterian Hospital, 520 East 70th Street, K415, NY 10021, USA
* Corresponding author.
*E-mail address:* jkm2001@med.cornell.edu (J.K. Min).

Cardiol Clin 27 (2009) 573–585
doi:10.1016/j.ccl.2009.06.005
0733-8651/09/$ – see front matter 

treadmill scores, and higher summed stress scores (**Fig. 1**).

Nevertheless, discordance between anatomic measures of intraluminal stenosis severity and functional perfusion—already well described in the ICA literature—may be anticipated by CCTA as well. Schuijf and colleagues[8] observed among 114 patients undergoing both MPS and CCTA that, while 90% of patients with no visualized plaque by CCTA had normal MPS, only 45% with any plaque by CCTA had abnormal MPS, and only 50% with any greater than 50% plaque by CCTA had abnormal MPS. However, among a subset subsequently sent to ICA, agreement between ICA and CCTA was high at 90%, while agreement between invasive angiography and MPS was much lower at 64%. Gaemperli and colleagues[9] characterized among 78 patients the diagnostic properties of greater than 50% disease identified by CCTA for MPS-identified ischemia, with a sensitivity, specificity, NPV, and PPV of 95%, 53%, 94%, and 58%, respectively on a per-patient basis, and 95%, 75%, 96%, and 72%, respectively, on a per-artery basis. Again, these discordances between CCTA obstructive plaque and MPS-identified ischemia were also observed with quantitative coronary angiography (QCA), with similar area under curve (AUC) [0.88 (0.80–0.96) for CCTA, 0.87 (0.79–0.94) for QCA] and with identical probabilities of ischemic detection by CCTA and QCA percent-diameter stenoses. From these data, investigators have argued that MPS and CCTA may provide discrete and potentially complementary information related to coronary artery disease (CAD)—that is, detection of myocardial ischemia and detection of coronary atherosclerosis.

## PROGNOSTIC VALUE OF CCTA FOR EVALUATION OF STABLE CHEST-PAIN SYNDROMES

As intraluminal stenosis by ICA and calcified plaque burden by coronary calcium scoring have both been well characterized for their prognostic value to predict incident CAD events, a reasonable hypothesis might posit that contrast-enhanced CCTA to visualize both intraluminal and extraluminal disease should provide greater discrimination for later cardiac events. In recent years, studies examining this risk-predictive ability have been an area of active interest. A summary of the available prognostic data on CCTA is summarized in **Table 1A** and **B**.

Given the relatively recent introduction of 64-slice CCTA, the earliest prognostic data relies upon older generations of CCTA scanners. The authors have reported the all-cause mortality of a single-center cohort of 1,127 low- to intermediate-risk symptomatic patients undergoing 16-slice CCTA for diagnosis of stable chest-pain syndromes over an intermediate-term observation period averaging 15 plus or minus 3.9 months.[10] CCTA scans were visually assessed for minimal or absent (<30% stenosis, score = 0), mild (30%–49%, score = 1), moderate (50%–69%, score = 2), or severe (>70% stenosis, score = 3) over a 16-segment modified American Heart Association model. Intraluminal stenosis severity predicted increased risk of death, with obstructions greater than or equal to 50% and greater than or equal to 70%, each portending worse prognosis. Proximity of disease, particularly in the left main (LM) or proximal left anterior descending (LAD) artery, and the vascular distribution of disease, as described by the number of epicardial vessels

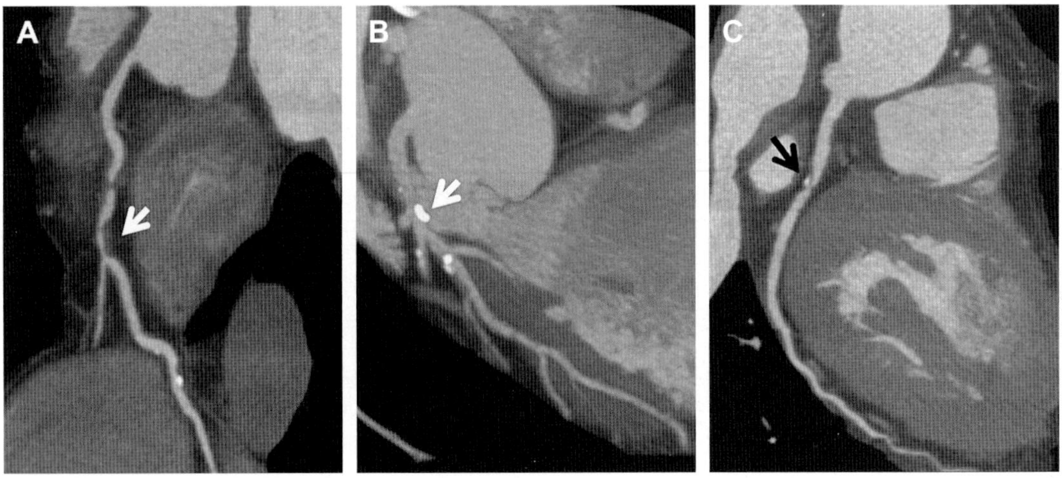


**Fig. 1.** Oblique maximum intensity projection CCTA images, with arrows demonstrating (*A*) noncalcified, (*B*) calcified, and (*C*) mixed plaque as visualized by CT angiography.

**Table 1A**
**Summary of prognostic data for CCTA**

| Study | Technology | Patient Population | | Follow up | Endpoint | | | | |
|---|---|---|---|---|---|---|---|---|---|
| | | Known CAD | No Known CAD | | ACM | Cardiac Death | MI | USA | TVR |
| Min et al[10] | 16-slice CT | *n* = 1,127, suspected CAD | | 15.3 ± 3.9 months | × | | | | |
| Pundziute et al[11] | 16- and 64-slice CT | *n* = 65 (65%) | *n* = 35 (35%) | 16 months (mean) | | × | × | × | × |
| Gaemperli et al[12] | 64-slice CT | *n* = 37 (17%) | *n* = 183 (83%) | 14 ± 4 months | | × | × | × | × |
| Van Werkhoven et al[13] | 16- and 64-slice CT | *n* = 517, suspected CAD | | 672 days (median) | × | | × | × | × |
| Ostrom et al[14] | EBCT | *n* = 2,538, suspected CAD | | 6.5 years (mean) | × | | | | |
| Hoffman et al[15] | 64-slice CT | *n* = 10 (9.7%) | *n* = 93 (90.3%) | 5 months | | × | × | × | × |
| Choi et al[22] | 64-slice CT | *n* = 1,000, asymptomatic | | 17 ± 2 months | | × | | × | × |
| Matsumoto et al[24] | 4- and 16-slice CT | *n* = 57 (7%) | *n* = 753 (93%) | 35 ± 18 months | | × | × | × | |
| Cademartiri et al[25] | 64-slice CT | *n* = 46 (47%) | *n* = 52 (53%) | 25 (mean) | | × | × | × | × |

*Abbreviations:* ACM, All-cause mortality; CAD, Coronary artery disease; MI, Myocardial infarction; TVR, Target vessel revascularization; USA, Unstable angina.

**Table 1B**
**Summary of prognostic data for CCTA**

| | | | | | Event Rate - No. of patients in category, percent-reached endpoint, HR(CI) | | | | | |
|---|---|---|---|---|---|---|---|---|---|---|
| | | | | | Vessels with obstructive CAD | | | | | |
| Study | No CAD | Nonobstructive CAD (≤50% stenosis) | Obstructive CAD (≥50% stenosis) | Any CAD | 1 Vessel | 2 Vessels | 3 Vessels | LM/LAD | Any proximal disease | No. of segments involved (HR is per segment) |
| Min et al[10] | ($n$ = 333) 0.3% | | | ($n$ = 794) 4.8% | | | Any severity HR 2.0(0.99–4.2) $P$ = .05 | LM only, any stenosis ($n$ = 176) 15% HR 2.7(1.4–5.1) $P \leq .0001$ | HR 1.4(0.7–2.8) NS | HR 1.16 (1.05–1.28) $P$ = .004 |
| Pundziute et al[11] | ($n$ = 20) 0% | ($n$ = 48) 8% HR 2.7(0.32–22) $P$ = .36 (NS) | ($n$ = 32) 63% HR 22(2.9–166) $P$ = .003 | ($n$ = 80) 30% HR 8.8(1.1–70) $P$ = .04 | | | | ($n$ = 23) 77% HR 36(4.7–276) $P$ = .0006 | | Any plaque: HR 1.3(1.1–1.4) $P$ = .0005 obstructive plaque: HR 1.8(1.5–2.1) $P$<.0001 mixed plaque: HR 1.5(1.3–1.9) $P$ = .0002 |
| Gaemperli et al[12] | ($n$ = 43) 0% | ($n$ = 125) 3% | ($n$ = 95) 59% HR 12.7(2.6–61.7) $P$ = .002 | ($n$ = 177) 34% HR 30(2.2–420.1) $P$ = .011 | ($n$ = 40) 50% | ($n$ = 39) 62% | ($n$ = 16) 75% | ($n$ = 76) 62% HR 10.4(5.5–19.8) $P$<.001 | ($n$ = 75) 55% HR 7.5(2.3–24) $P$ = .001 | HR 1.3(1.2–1.4) $P$<.001 |
| Van Werkhoven et al[13] | ($n$ = 155) 1.1% annually | ($n$ = 204) 2% annually | ($n$ = 158) 6.3% annually HR 3.68(1.62–8.42) $P$ = .002 | ($n$ = 362) HR 3.09(0.92–10.39) NS | | | | | | Other findings—≥2 Noncalcified plaques: ($n$ = 65) 8.4% annually HR 5(2.2–11.7%) No/mild CAD and nl MPS 1% annually No/mild CAD and + MPS 3.7% annually > 50% stenosis and nl MPS 3.8% annually > 50% stenosis and + MPS 9% annually |
| Ostrom et al[14] | ($n$ = 1085) 1.7% | | | ($n$ = 1,453) 4.7% HR 2.7 (1.6–4.5) $P$ = .0001 | ($n$ = 310) 7.1% HR 1.8(1.4–2.5) $P$ = .0001 Nonobstruc-tive: ($n$ = 750) 2.7% HR 1.03(0.3–1.7) NS | ($n$ = 68) 11.3% HR 2.3(1.9–2.9) $P$ = .0001 Nonobstruc-tive: ($n$ = 238) 4.6% HR 1.02(0.68–1.9) NS | ($n$ = 15) 20% HR 2.6(2–3.4) $P$ = .0001 Nonobstruc-tive: ($n$ = 72) 6.9% HR 1.7(1.3–2.3) $P$ = .0001 | | | |
| Hoffman et al[15] | ($n$ = 41) NPV 100% | ($n$ = 32) | ($n$ = 30) Sensitivity 77% Specificity 87% NPV 98% PPV 35% | ($n$ = 62) Sensitivity 100% Specificity 54% NPV 100% PPV 17% | | | | | | |

| | | | | |
|---|---|---|---|---|
| Choi et al[22] | ($n$ = 785) 0% | | ($n$ = 215) 7% | Noncalcified plaque: ($n$ = 40) 5% rate of MACE |
| Matsumoto et al[24] | | | | Nonobstructive noncalc-ified plaques: ($n$ = 189) MI 2.64% USA 2.64% Death 1.05% OR 2.53(1.08–5.92) $P$<.05 Nonobstruc-tive mixed or calcified plaques: ($n$ = 621) MI 0.32% USA 1.61% Death 0.64% |
| Cademartiri et al[25] | +DM: ($n$ = 3) 0% −DM: ($n$ = 10) 0% | +DM: ($n$ = 17) 5.9% −DM: ($n$ = ) 0% | +DM: ($n$ = 25) 51.7%, $P$ = .003 −DM: ($n$ = 20) 42.1%, $P$ = .0004 | |

*Abbreviations:* CAD, Coronary artery disease; DM, Diabetes mellitus; HR, Hazard ratio; MACE, Major adverse cardiac events; MI, Myocardial infarction.

involved, also portended worse prognosis ($P<.001$). Finally, the extent and distribution of disease predicted risk in a graded fashion. The modified Duke CAD jeopardy score adapted from ICA, integrating disease extent, proximal distribution, and LM disease, discriminated risk among patients by higher-risk Duke scores, ranging from 96% survival for one stenosis greater than or equal to 70% or two stenoses greater than or equal to 50% ($P = .013$ compared with no disease) to 85% survival for greater than or equal to 50% LM artery stenosis ($P<.0001$). Simple scores to characterize plaque burden, such as the segment-involvement score (summating plaque presence over 16 segments) and the segment-stenosis score (summating plaque ratings over 16 segments, for a maximum of 45) predicted 5% to 6% higher absolute death rate for scores greater than 5 (6.6% versus 1.6% and 8.4% versus 2.5%, respectively; $P = .05$ for both). In patients with no evident disease in any coronary artery, in the LM artery or in the proximal LAD artery, the NPV for death by all causes in a 15-month follow-up were 99.7%, 97.8%, and 98.4%, respectively, revealing that a negative CCTA predicts a good prognosis.

The near- to intermediate-term prognostic value of CCTA in the stable chest-pain population has also been characterized for major adverse cardiac events (MACE). Pundziute and colleagues[11] studied 100 patients with known or suspected significant CAD who had undergone 16- or 64-slice CCTA, with 33 MACE events among 26 patients (unstable angina, myocardial infarction, death, and coronary revascularization) over a mean follow-up of 16 months. Patients with normal coronary arteries by multislice computed tomography had a 1-year event rate of 0%, while those with obstructive greater than or equal to 50% disease had significantly elevated event rates (63%), particularly if lesions were located in the LM or LAD artery (77%). Obstructive CAD (HR 22, confidence interval or CI 2.9–166, $P = .003$), and obstructive LM/LAD disease (HR 36, CI 4.7–276, $P = .0006$) were independent predictors of events in multivariate analysis over baseline clinical risk factors. Among the patients with obstructive disease, the event rate was driven primarily by early revascularization, which may have been increased by the depiction of obstructive disease in this open-label study. However, even patients with nonobstructive (<50%) disease had an elevated risk of MACE events of 8%, which could not be explained by early revascularization. Additionally, the number of segments with "mixed" plaques was also an independent predictor of MACE events, while the number of segments with calcified plaques did not, supporting the concept that detection and characterization of extraluminal disease will provide additional prognostic information beyond intraluminal stenosis alone.

Gaemperli and colleagues[12] studied the predictive value for MACE events with 64-slice CCTA exclusively in a larger cohort of 220 patients with known or suspected CAD who underwent 64-slice CCTA. Over 14 plus or minus 4 months, 27% had MACE events, comparable to the Pundziute cohort. Those with no detectable CAD had an event rate of 0%, while those with abnormal coronaries had an overall rate of 34%, with significantly more events seen in obstructive disease ($\geq$50% stenosis) at a first-year event rate of 59%. In addition, the investigators noted that events increased with the number of vessels involved, but the strongest association was found with LM, LAD, and any proximal epicardial vessel disease, concordant with earlier studies. In multivariate analysis, only obstructive CAD conferred independent increase in risk [HR, 12.65 (95% CI, 2.59–61.72); $P = .002$]. Again, in this open-label trial, event rates were primarily driven by early revascularization, while death, unstable angina, and myocardial infarction were not significant alone. In receiver-operator curve analysis, the optimal threshold for identification of increased risk appeared to occur in the presence of three or more individual plaques with at least one obstructive stenosis in any distribution, suggesting that there may be a CCTA-identifiable threshold for initiation of aggressive medical therapy.

To assess the predictive value of CCTA for late events exclusive of revascularization, and to evaluate the relative prognostic performance of MPS and CCTA, van Werkhoven and colleagues[13] conducted a multicenter study of 541 intermediate probability patients referred for symptoms or CAD risk factors who prospectively underwent both CCTA and MPS. Similar to previous results, half of the patients with at least one greater than or equal to 50% stenosis by CCTA had abnormal MPS with a summed stress score greater than or equal to 4, while only half of the patients with abnormal MPS had abnormal CCTA. Interestingly, of those with normal MPS, 22% had a greater than or equal to 50% lesion by CCTA. Excluding patients who underwent early revascularization within 60 days of imaging, of the 439 patients followed over a median of 672 days (interquartile range 420–896), 23 patients (5.2%) had myocardial infarction, death, or unstable angina requiring revascularization. The annualized hard event rate was 1.8% in those with none or mild CAD versus 4.8% in those with greater than or equal to 50% stenosis by CCTA, and 1.1% in those with a normal versus 3.8% in those with an abnormal MPS. In multivariate analysis, CCTA-visualized obstructive plaque and abnormal MPS were independent predictors of late events after adjustment for clinical risk factors, with significantly improved prediction by combined use of CCTA and myocardial perfusion imaging compared with either modality alone (log-rank test *P*-value <0.005). The presence of more than two noncalcified plaques additionally improved prediction of risk beyond CCTA obstructive disease and MPS alone, supporting a continued value to visualization of extraluminal plaque. Over the study period, those with concordantly normal CCTA and MPS had an annualized hard event rate of 1%, those with concordantly abnormal CCTA and MPS had a hard event rate of 9.0%, and those with discordant CCTA and MPS with either abnormal CCTA or abnormal MPS had event rates of 3.8% and 3.7%, respectively. Those with no visualized plaque by CCTA had the best prognosis, with a hard event rate of 0.3%. This study supports the complementary diagnostic and prognostic value of CCTA and MPS, as well as the prognostic value of extraluminal plaque. It is interesting that noncalcified plaque in this cohort was a significant predictor of late events, while mixed plaque predicted late events in other cohorts. One potential explanation lies in differences between study populations, as those patients who underwent early revascularization and provided the majority of events in the Gaemperli and Pundziute study populations were excluded from this cohort, pointing out a difference in predictors of near- and long-term events, as well as revascularization versus other cardiac outcomes.

As 64-slice multidetector CT scanners have not been clinically available for a sufficient duration for accumulation of observation beyond 2 to 3 years, the long-term prognostic performance of CCTA must be extrapolated from electron-beam tomography, with a lesser spatial resolution compared with present day technology. Ostrom and colleagues[14] studied the all-cause mortality of 2,538 consecutive symptomatic patients without known CAD over an observation period averaging 6.5 years, with 86 deaths observed. Patients with no visualized plaques had an excellent survival of 98.3%, while those with any diagnosed CAD had a threefold greater mortality with a survival of 95.3% (**Fig. 2**). The extent and severity of plaque predicted all-cause mortality in a graded fashion, by the extent and severity of disease, with significantly elevated hazards seen not only for three-vessel, two-vessel, and one-vessel obstructive (≥50%) disease [adjusted HR (95% CI) 2.59 (1.99–3.68), 2.31 (1.86–2.89), 1.82 (1.45–2.3) respectively], but also for three-vessel nonobstructive disease [1.74 (1.49–2.05)], nearly equal to the risks in single-vessel obstructive disease (**Fig. 3**). Angiographic disease by electron-beam CTA significantly improved

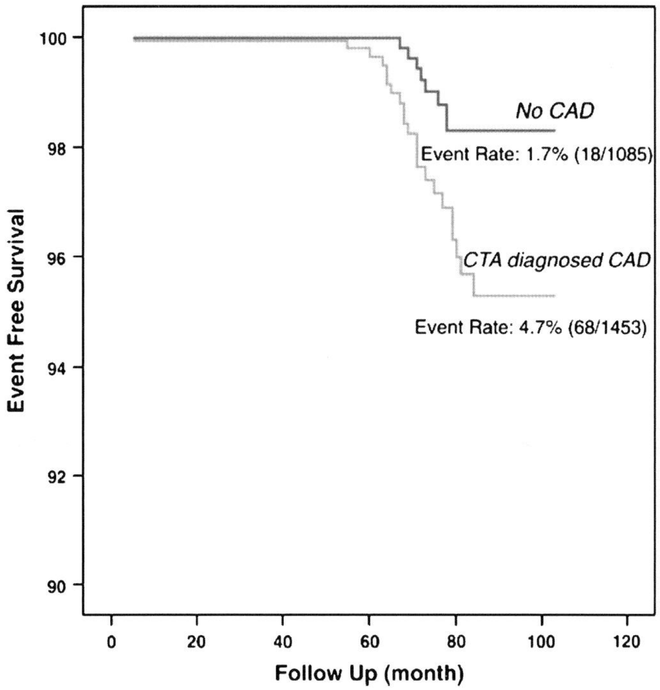


**Fig. 2.** Risk-adjusted event-free survival according to extent of CCTA-diagnosed CAD (*Reprinted from* Ostrom MP, Gopal A, Ahmadi N, et al. Mortality incidence and the severity of coronary atherosclerosis assessed by computed tomography angiography. J Am Coll Cardiol 2008;52(16):1338.).

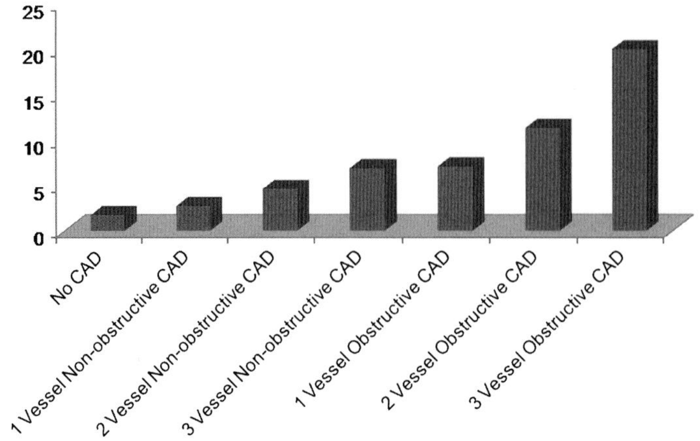


**Fig. 3.** Progressive extent and severity of CCTA-diagnosed CAD correlate with increasing all-cause mortality. (*Data from* Ostrom MP, Gopal A, Ahmadi N, et al. Mortality incidence and the severity of coronary atherosclerosis assessed by computed tomography angiography. J Am Coll Cardiol 2008;52(16):1339.)

incremental prognostic power compared with traditional risk-factor assessment alone [AUC 0.83 (0.77–0.88) compared with 0.69 (0.61-0.77), $P = .0001$]. Additionally, calcium score was independently predictive after accounting for risk factors and angiographic disease, suggesting a continued role for characterization of global-plaque burden and composition. In the future, 64-slice CCTA, with diagnostic performance superior to electron-beam CT, should perform as well or better for long-term prognosis.

## PROGNOSTIC VALUE OF CCTA IN ACUTE CORONARY SYNDROMES

CCTA has been investigated as an alternative diagnostic modality for acute chest pain evaluation in several studies.[15–20] Hoffmann and colleagues[15] first observed in a single-center, double-blinded cohort of 103 patients with initially negative troponin and electrocardiograms for in-hospital and 6-month outcomes of acute coronary syndrome (ACS) diagnosis and major adverse cardiac events. Eight percent of the patients developed ACS during the hospitalization and 0% had any cardiac events; of the ACS patients, 7 out of 31 had nonobstructive plaque by CCTA, but none had no plaque at all. Using the triage criterion of either any plaque or greater than 50% stenosis, the sensitivities were 100% and 77%, the specificities were 54% and 87%, the NPVs were 100% and 98%, and the PPVs were 17% and 35%, respectively. In this patient population, the absence of any CAD on CCTA would have allowed for early safe discharge for 50% of the patients, and the AUC for the presence of stenosis was 0.82, as compared with the AUC for the Thrombolysis In Myocardial Infarction (TIMI) risk score of 0.63. However, the low PPV of CCTA underscores the findings that a 50% threshold for intraluminal coronary artery stenosis is an imperfect metric for the identification of ACS.

Other investigators studying a wide range of disease prevalences from 0% to 34% have found high NPVs for CCTA-visualized obstructive stenosis for prediction of ACS and near-term MACE events, with ranges of NPVs of 97% to 100%, depending upon the pretest probability of disease.[17–19] Goldstein and colleagues[16] performed a randomized controlled trial comparing rest MPS to CCTA in a low-risk cohort of 197 ACS patients with negative serial troponin measurements, and found identically low event rates over 6 months of follow-up of 0%, with earlier discharge and lower costs observed in the CCTA group ($P<.001$).

In the larger multicenter double-blinded ROMICAT study, Hoffman and colleagues[21] observed 368 patients presenting to the emergency department with acute chest pain who underwent 64-slice CCTA after initially negative troponin measurements and electrocardiograms. None of the 185 patients with no visualized CAD had ACS, while 7 of the 115 with nonobstructive plaque and 24 of the 68 with significant obstructive or nondiagnostic examinations had ACS during the index hospitalization; there were 0 MACE during 6-month follow-up. This resulted in a NPV of 100% for any plaque and 98% for greater than 50% stenosis for 6-month MACE events, inclusive of in-hospital diagnosis of ACS. Additionally, CCTA incrementally improved prediction of ACS beyond the TIMI risk score, with an AUC for CCTA-visualized extent of plaque 0.88 and CCTA-visualized stenotic disease of 0.82, compared with the AUC of the TIMI risk score of 0.63. In aggregate, the current data on CCTA for ACS suggests that in the appropriate populations, CCTA-visualized abnormalities provides risk stratification for near-term events, and that a 100% NPV for the triage criterion of the presence of any plaque may allow for safe, early discharge in a large proportion of low-risk ACS patients. On the other hand, the presence of nonobstructive coronary artery plaque portends a low but nonzero risk, congruent with the data observed in the chronic chest pain population, and is therefore an imperfect triage criteria for ACS.

## PROGNOSTIC VALUE OF CCTA FOR ASYMPTOMATIC PATIENTS

Given the prognostic value of coronary calcium scoring for risk stratification in asymptomatic patients, it is reasonable that atherosclerosis visualization with CCTA should have prognostic value in asymptomatic patients as well, although it is unclear if the risk-benefit ratio among asymptomatic patients justifies the use of CCTA. Choi and colleagues[22] studied 1,000 asymptomatic patients who underwent 64-slice CCTA as part of a general health evaluation. As might be expected, the prevalence of severe ($\geq$75% stenosis) disease was low at only 2%. Those with no plaque had no major adverse cardiac events over an average observation of 17 plus or minus 2 months, while 15 of the 215 individuals with any plaque had later unstable angina or underwent revascularization. Most events occurred within 90 days of the CCTA and were driven by revascularization procedures in this open-label trial. From these data, it appears that although the prevalence of occult CAD in these apparently healthy middle-aged individuals was not negligible, and that CCTA findings may provide a limited measure of risk stratification, the intermediate prognosis—even among those with occult CAD—was good and did not justify use of CCTA for population-based screening.

## PROGNOSTIC VALUE OF EXTRALUMINAL PLAQUE VISUALIZATION BY CCTA

CCTA noninvasive depiction of extraluminal coronary plaque, otherwise feasible only with invasive means such as intravascular ultrasound, enhances prediction of later events in multiple studies, as already described. CCTA enhances detection of nonobstructive plaques, which are equally likely to give rise to ACS as obstructive stenoses, and assists in differentiation between calcified, noncalcified, and mixed lesions, although the overlap in Hounsfield units does not permit differentiation between lipid-laden and fibrous lesions.[23] Matsumoto and colleagues[24] observed 810 patients with nonobstructive coronary artery disease for ACS and cardiac death over 35 plus or minus 18 months for ACS or cardiac death. The 22% of patients with at least one low-density plaque (Hounsfield unit density < 68 HU) had elevated rates of ACS and cardiac death (5.29% and 1.05% respectively) compared with those without low-density plaques (1.93% and 0.64%, respectively, $P<.001$ for ACS and $P$ = NS for cardiac death). In multivariate analysis, among patients with nonobstructive plaques, only previous myocardial infarction and the presence of low-density plaques predicted later ACS [HR 2.53 (1.08-5.92), $P<.05$]. These findings underscore the risks presented by plaques that would not have been detected by calcium scoring or ischemia testing, and also the differential transformative potential of atherosclerotic plaques by composition.

## PROGNOSTIC VALUE OF CCTA IN SELECT SUBPOPULATIONS

Cademartiri and colleagues[25] examined the prognostic value of CCTA among 49 patients with and 49 without diabetes over 20 months. Atherosclerotic plaques, and especially significant stenoses greater than 50%, were more prevalent in the diabetic population ($P$ = .02); only 6.1% of the diabetics had absence of any plaque by CCTA. Among both groups, the presence of significant CAD on CCTA predicted death, nonfatal myocardial infarction, or hospitalization for unstable angina, increasing with the degree of obstruction ($P<.01$ for both groups). Among both diabetics and nondiabetics, the absence of any visualized atherosclerosis predicted an excellent prognosis, with zero events in both groups, while diabetics with CCTA-defined nonobstructive or obstructive CAD had a higher risk of later events compared with nondiabetics (5.9% versus 0% and 51.7% versus 42%, respectively). Concordant with the MPS literature, diabetics with "nonsignificant" scans, as defined by the presence of nonobstructive lesions, have a lesser warranty period for later events than nondiabetics; however, unlike MPS, CCTA is able to define a small cohort of diabetics with an excellent prognosis comparable to nondiabetics, because MPS cannot differentiate patients with mild disease from those with normal coronaries. The prognostic value of CCTA for other special populations, such as women or ethnic minorities, has not yet been defined, although long-term studies as proposed for the Multi-Ethnic

Study of Atherosclerosis Computed Tomography substudy will address these important questions in the future.

## PROGNOSTIC VALUE OF NONCORONARY FINDINGS BY CCTA

As CCTA is able to image all structures in three dimensions throughout the cardiac cycle, it can accurately characterize multiple noncoronary findings, such as pulmonary veins, left ventricular mass, congenital diseases, masses, aortic or valvular abnormalities, and provide a functional assessment in the form of ejection fraction.[26,27] While CCTA has been evaluated for its diagnostic accuracy for cardiac structure and function—including ventricular and atrial volume measures, valvular regurgitation and stenosis, and aortic atherosclerosis—the prognostic interpretation of these measures by CCTA have not yet been comprehensively performed. Indeed, only recently have age- and gender-specific normative reference values for the heart and great vessels by CCTA been developed.[28] These and other findings with prognostic value established by echocardiography and invasive angiography, such as left ventricular function, mass and geometry, and left atrial volume and size, may add predictive value beyond coronary arteries regarding comprehensive risk of incident MACE (**Fig. 4**).

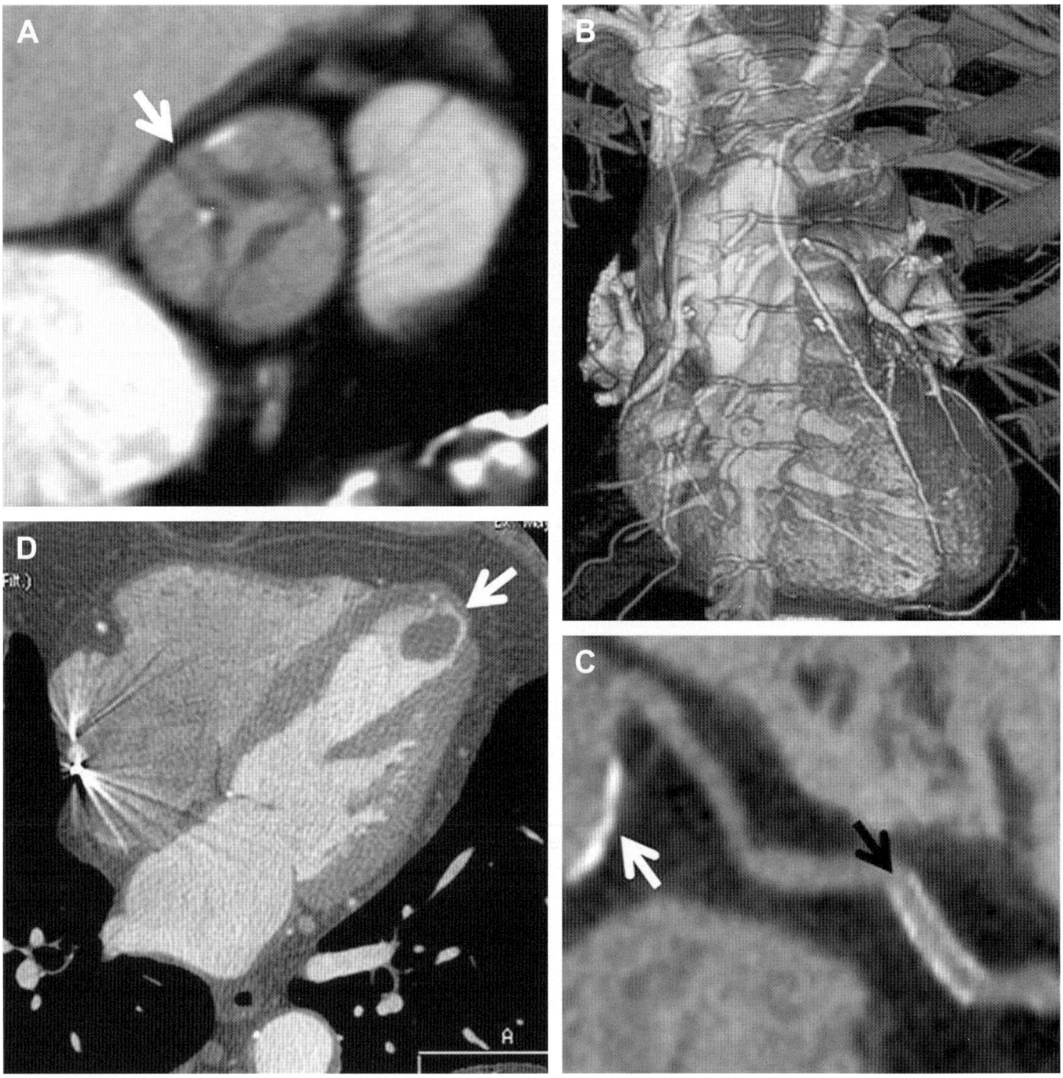


**Fig. 4.** Other findings by CCTA. Coronary CT angiography provides information beyond coronary artery atherosclerosis such as visualization of (*A*) the number and calcification (*arrow*) of aortic valve leaflets, (*B*) coronary artery bypass grafts, (*C*) intracoronary stents (*black arrow*) and aortic atherosclerosis (*white arrow*), and (*D*) left ventricular thrombus (*arrow*).

## SAFETY AND APPROPRIATENESS OF CCTA FOR RISK STRATIFICATION

Technologic limitations of current-generation CCTA scanners result in stenosis estimates at one-third the spatial resolution of ICA, with a spatial resolution of 0.625 mm, precluding the accurate evaluation of small arteries below 2 mm; beam-hardening artifacts generated by metallic or heavily calcified structures will also limit the diagnostic accuracy of CCTA. Current-generation scanners also require a 5- to 10-second breath-hold and slow, regular heart rates ideally less than 70 beats per minute to capture still frames of the small, rapidly moving coronary arteries, and dye loads of 60 mL to 80 mL of iodinated contrast, requiring selection of patients without arrhythmias, renal insufficiency, or inability to breath-hold who would be able to undergo studies of sufficient diagnostic quality for analysis. Finally, although most of the studies reviewed in this article include some proportion of patients with prior CAD, none included solely patients with prior revascularization, precluding generalization of those findings to patients with stents or bypass grafts.

The risks and benefits of the additional risk stratification to be gained by CCTA must be weighed for different groups of patients with consideration of pretest probability. In a large statewide registry, Raff and colleagues[29] found that the median radiation dose for CCTA was 25.0 mSv (25%–75% range, 15 mSv–30 mSv). However, Hausleiter and colleagues[30] found in the PROTECTION-1 study, a large international registry of 1,965 patients in 50 sites, a lower estimated median dose of 12.0 mSv (interquartile range 7.4 mSv–17 mSv), with lower doses independently predicted by lower patient weight, scan length, use of 100-kV tube voltage, presence of stable sinus rhythm, use of dose modulation over the cardiac cycle, and scanning-center volume and experience. Using prospective gating to limit overlap of radiation coverage and reduce exposure throughout the cardiac cycle in combination with the aforementioned dose-reduction techniques can result in doses as low as 1.2 mSv without reductions in image quality.[31,32] Current guidelines, established before the majority of the studies described in this review, cover only diagnostic uses of CCTA but should address the appropriateness of risk stratification in different populations, as radiation reduction protocols and prognostic data for CCTA emerge.[2,33,34]

## SUMMARY

The severity, location, and extent of CAD as detected by CCTA have prognostic value for near- and long-term prediction of major adverse cardiac events, as well as the hard endpoint of all-cause mortality. Abnormalities by CCTA are both predictive of and complementary to abnormalities by MPS for diagnosis and prognosis of CAD, reflecting the differing pathophysiology underlying anatomic and functional disease. Normal CCTAs, in particular those with no evident coronary artery plaque, portend an excellent prognosis, while those with nonobstructive plaques have a low but nonzero risk of later events, particularly in diabetics and patients presenting with acute coronary syndromes, even among asymptomatic patients. Enhanced detection of nonobstructive CAD and extraluminal plaque composition has additive predictive value beyond characterization of the coronary arterial lumen alone. Future studies and appropriateness guidelines addressing different subpopulations, treatment strategies based upon CCTA findings, and incorporating aggregate measures of coronary luminal stenosis, extraluminal plaque composition, and noncoronary cardiac findings will help to define the clinical role of risk stratification of CCTA for patient management.

## REFERENCES


1. Budoff MJ, Dowe D, Jollis JG, et al. Diagnostic performance of 64-multidetector row coronary computed tomographic angiography for evaluation of coronary artery stenosis in individuals without known coronary artery disease: results from the prospective multicenter ACCURACY (Assessment by Coronary Computed Tomographic Angiography of Individuals Undergoing Invasive Coronary Angiography) trial. J Am Coll Cardiol 2008;52(21): 1724–32.
2. Fraker TD Jr, Fihn SD, Chronic Stable Angina Writing Committee, et al. 2007 chronic angina focused update of the ACC/AHA 2002 guidelines for the management of patients with chronic stable angina: a report of the American College of Cardiology/American Heart Association Task Force on Practice Guidelines Writing Group to develop the focused update of the 2002 guidelines for the management of patients with chronic stable angina. J Am Coll Cardiol 2007;50(23):2264–74.
3. Brindis RG, Douglas PS, Hendel RC, et al. American College of Cardiology Foundation Quality Strategic Directions Committee Appropriateness Criteria Working Group; American Society of Nuclear Cardiology; American Heart Association. ACCF/ASNC appropriateness criteria for single-photon emission computed tomography myocardial perfusion imaging (SPECT MPI): a report of the American College of Cardiology Foundation Quality Strategic

Directions Committee Appropriateness Criteria Working Group and the American Society of Nuclear Cardiology endorsed by the American Heart Association. J Am Coll Cardiol 2005;46(8):1587–605.
4. Miller JM, Rochitte CE, Dewey M, et al. Diagnostic performance of coronary angiography by 64-row CT. N Engl J Med 2008;359(22):2324–36.
5. Meijboom WB, Meijs MF, Schuijf JD, et al. Diagnostic accuracy of 64-slice computed tomography coronary angiography: a prospective, multicenter, multivendor study. J Am Coll Cardiol 2008;52(25):2135–44.
6. Lin FY, Saba S, Weinsaft JW, et al. Relation of plaque characteristics defined by coronary computed tomographic angiography to ST-segment depression and impaired functional capacity during exercise treadmill testing in patients suspected of having coronary heart disease. Am J Cardiol 2009;103(1):50–8.
7. Lin F, Shaw LJ, Berman DS, et al. Multidetector computed tomography coronary artery plaque predictors of stress-induced myocardial ischemia by SPECT. Atherosclerosis 2008;197(2):700–9.
8. Schuijf JD, Wijns W, Jukema JW, et al. Relationship between noninvasive coronary angiography with multi-slice computed tomography and myocardial perfusion imaging. J Am Coll Cardiol 2006;48(12):2508–14.
9. Gaemperli O, Schepis T, Valenta I, et al. Functionally relevant coronary artery disease: comparison of 64-section CT angiography with myocardial perfusion SPECT. Radiology 2008;248(2):414–23.
10. Min JK, Shaw LJ, Devereux RB, et al. Prognostic value of multidetector coronary computed tomographic angiography for prediction of all-cause mortality. J Am Coll Cardiol 2007;50(12):1161–70.
11. Pundziute G, Schuijf JD, Jukema JW, et al. Prognostic value of multislice computed tomography coronary angiography in patients with known or suspected coronary artery disease. J Am Coll Cardiol 2007;49(1):62–70.
12. Gaemperli O, Valenta I, Schepis T, et al. Coronary 64-slice CT angiography predicts outcome in patients with known or suspected coronary artery disease. Eur Radiol 2008;18:1162–73.
13. van Werkhoven JM, Schuijf JD, Gaemperli O, et al. Prognostic value of multislice computed tomography and gated single-photon emission computed tomography in patients with suspected coronary artery disease. J Am Coll Cardiol 2009;53(7):623–32.
14. Ostrom MP, Gopal A, Ahmadi N, et al. Mortality incidence and the severity of coronary atherosclerosis assessed by computed tomography angiography. J Am Coll Cardiol 2008;52(16):1335–43.
15. Hoffmann U, Nagurney JT, Moselewski F, et al. Coronary multidetector computed tomography in the assessment of patients with acute chest pain. Circulation 2006;114(21):2251–60.
16. Goldstein JA, Gallagher MJ, O'Neill WW, et al. A randomized controlled trial of multi-slice coronary computed tomography for evaluation of acute chest pain. J Am Coll Cardiol 2007;49(8):863–71.
17. Rubinshtein R, Halon DA, Gaspar T, et al. Usefulness of 64-slice cardiac computed tomographic angiography for diagnosing acute coronary syndromes and predicting clinical outcome in emergency department patients with chest pain of uncertain origin. Circulation 2007;115(13):1762–8.
18. Gallagher MJ, Ross MA, Raff GL, et al. The diagnostic accuracy of 64-slice computed tomography coronary angiography compared with stress nuclear imaging in emergency department low-risk chest pain patients. Ann Emerg Med 2007;49(2):125–36.
19. Hollander JE, Litt HI, Chase M, et al. Computed tomography coronary angiography for rapid disposition of low-risk emergency department patients with chest pain syndromes. Acad Emerg Med 2007;14(2):112–6.
20. Noda M, Takagi A, Kuwatsuru R, et al. Prognostic significance of multi-detector computed tomography in conjunction with TIMI risk score for patients with acute coronary syndrome. Heart Vessels 2008;23:161–6.
21. Hoffmann U, Bamberg F, Chae CU, et al. Coronary computed tomography angiography for early triage of patients with acute chest pain: the Rule Out Myocardial Infarction using Computer Assisted Tomography (ROMICAT) trial. J Am Coll Cardiol 2009;53(18):1642–50.
22. Choi EK, Choi SI, Rivera JJ, et al. Coronary computed tomography angiography as a screening tool for the detection of occult coronary artery disease in asymptomatic individuals. J Am Coll Cardiol 2008;52(5):357–65.
23. Leber AW, Knez A, Becker A, et al. Accuracy of multidetector spiral computed tomography in identifying and differentiating the composition of coronary atherosclerotic plaques: a comparative study with intracoronary ultrasound. J Am Coll Cardiol 2004;43(7):1241–7.
24. Matsumoto N, Sato Y, Yoda S, et al. Prognostic value of non-obstructive CT low-dense coronary artery plaques detected by multislice computed tomography. Circ J 2007;71(12):1898–903.
25. Cademartiri F, Seitun S, Romano M, et al. Prognostic value of 64-slice coronary angiography in diabetes mellitus patients with known or suspected coronary artery disease compared with a nondiabetic population. Radiol Med 2008;113:627–43.
26. Sugeng L, Mor-Avi V, Weinert L, et al. Quantitative assessment of left ventricular size and function: side-by-side comparison of real-time three-dimensional echocardiography and computed tomography with magnetic resonance reference. Circulation 2006;114(7):654–61.
27. Belge B, Coche E, Pasquet A, et al. Accurate estimation of global and regional cardiac function by

retrospectively gated multidetector row computed tomography: comparison with cine magnetic resonance imaging. Eur Radiol 2006;16(7):1424–33.
28. Lin FY, Roman MJ, Meng J, et al. Cardiac chamber volumes, function and mass by 64-detector row computed tomography: age- and gender-specific values among healthy adults free of hypertension and obesity. JACC Cardiovasc Imaging 2008;1(6):782–6.
29. Raff GL, Chinnaiyan KM, Share DA, et al. Radiation dose from cardiac computed tomography before and after implementation of radiation dose-reduction techniques. JAMA 2009;301(22):2340–8.
30. Hausleiter J, Meyer T, Hermann F, et al. Estimated radiation dose associated with cardiac CT angiography. JAMA 2009;301(5):500–7.
31. Gopal A, Mao SS, Karlsberg D, et al. Radiation reduction with prospective ECG-triggering acquisition using 64-multidetector computed tomographic angiography. Int J Cardiovasc Imaging 2009;25(4):405–16.
32. Earls JP, Berman EL, Urban BA, et al. Prospectively gated transverse coronary CT angiography versus retrospectively gated helical technique: improved image quality and reduced radiation dose. Radiology 2008;246(3):742–53.
33. Hendel RC, Patel MR, Kramer CM, et al. American College of Cardiology Foundation Quality Strategic Directions Committee Appropriateness Criteria Working Group; American College of Radiology; Society of Cardiovascular Computed Tomography; Society for Cardiovascular Magnetic Resonance; American Society of Nuclear Cardiology; North American Society for Cardiac Imaging; Society for Cardiovascular Angiography and Interventions; Society of Interventional Radiology. ACCF/ACR/SCCT/SCMR/ASNC/NASCI/SCAI/SIR 2006 appropriateness criteria for cardiac computed tomography and cardiac magnetic resonance imaging. A report of the American College of Cardiology Foundation Quality Strategic Directions Committee Appropriateness Criteria Working Group. J Am Coll Cardiol 2006;48(7):1475–97.
34. Anderson JL, Adams CD, Antman EM, et al. ACC/AHA 2007 guidelines for the management of patients with unstable angina/non ST-elevation myocardial infarction: a report of the American College of Cardiology/American Heart Association Task Force on Practice Guidelines (Writing Committee to Revise the 2002 Guidelines for the Management of Patients With Unstable Angina/Non ST-Elevation Myocardial Infarction): developed in collaboration with the American College of Emergency Physicians, the Society for Cardiovascular Angiography and Interventions, and the Society of Thoracic Surgeons: endorsed by the American Association of Cardiovascular and Pulmonary Rehabilitation and the Society for Academic Emergency Medicine. Circulation 2007;116(7):e148–304.

# Cardiac CT in the Emergency Department

Kavitha M. Chinnaiyan, MD, FACC*, Gilbert L. Raff, MD, FACC, James A. Goldstein, MD, FACC

**KEYWORDS**

- Cardiac CT • Emergency department
- Acute chest pain • Acute coronary syndromes
- Coronary CT angiography

In the United States alone, nearly 6 million patients present annually to emergency departments (EDs) with complaints of chest pain suspicious for acute coronary ischemia.[1] Of these, approximately 75% of patients are found to have nonischemic cardiac (21%) or noncardiac (55%) problems. Of the remaining patients, 17% meet the criteria for acute cardiac ischemia, acute myocardial infarction (AMI; 8%), unstable angina (9%), or stable angina (6%).[2–4] High-risk patients with acute coronary syndrome(s) (ACS) are easily identified by the constellation of history, elevation in cardiac enzymes, and electrocardiographic (ECG) changes. On the other end of the spectrum, those with an extremely low probability of ACS can be discharged in an expedited fashion. A third group of patients, comprising those with a nonnegligible risk for ACS, undergo extended observation and workup for an ischemic cause. Of those admitted for extended observation, less than 30% of patients have true ACS.[2] Despite this approach, 2% to 8% of patients with ACS are misdiagnosed and inappropriately discharged home,[3,4] with a doubling of mortality associated with missed diagnosis of ACS.[4] Additionally, missed myocardial infarctions result in most malpractice suits against ED physicians.[5]

The serious consequences of diagnostic failure result in expensive time-consuming strategies to exclude ischemic etiologies of chest pain. In patients suspected of having ACS who lack ECG abnormalities and positive biomarkers on presentation, several protocols are used for conclusive evaluation. Some centers routinely admit these patients for extended observation, and others use dedicated short-stay "chest pain centers." Here, serial serum cardiac biomarkers and ECG are obtained to "rule-out myocardial infarction".[6–11] Usually, patients who have no evidence of ischemia by serial biomarkers and ECG undergo further risk stratification by stress testing. Rest myocardial perfusion imaging (with and without stress) with single-photon emission CT (SPECT) and stress echocardiography have been applied in this setting. Both modalities have been shown to provide incremental information for clinical risk stratification in these patients.[12–14] SPECT imaging is time-intensive, however, and stress echocardiography may fail to identify nontransmural infarcts.[15] Additionally, this approach of evaluation of patients who have acute chest pain with extended observation and ancillary testing incurs an estimated cost of $10 to $12 billion annually in this country alone.[1,6]

Importantly, although these current standard-of-care protocols are designed to detect physiologically significant coronary disease, information about the presence and extent of nonhemodynamically significant coronary artery disease (CAD) is not obtained, and a significant opportunity to commence aggressive preventive goals may be lost.

## ACCURACY OF CORONARY CT ANGIOGRAPHY COMPARED WITH INVASIVE ANGIOGRAPHY

Beginning with the introduction of four-slice spiral CT systems in 2000, rapid and revolutionary technologic advances in the spatial and temporal resolution of multislice CT have facilitated practical

Department of Cardiology, William Beaumont Hospital, 3601 West 13 Mile Road, Royal Oak, MI 48073, USA
* Corresponding author.
*E-mail address:* kchinnaiyan@beaumont.edu (K.M. Chinnaiyan).

Cardiol Clin 27 (2009) 587–596
doi:10.1016/j.ccl.2009.06.002
0733-8651/09/$ – see front matter 

coronary CT angiography (CCTA). The latest generation of 64-slice systems has reduced scan time to 5 to 10 seconds and has a spatial resolution of 0.4 mm, providing much wider anatomic coverage with each gantry rotation in addition to decreased breath-hold times and motion artifacts. Newer scanners with dual x-ray sources and detector arrays in the scanner gantry provide an additional 50% reduction in temporal resolution (ie, 83 milliseconds compared with 165 milliseconds in the 64-slice systems). A further decrease in acquisition times achieved with a single heartbeat is possible with new 256- and 320-slice scanners.[16,17]

The accuracy of CCTA for assessing the presence and severity of coronary atherosclerosis compared with invasive angiography has been reported in more than 30 published studies encompassing more than 2000 patients.[18–44] A meta-analysis of 29 studies (16- to 64-slice systems in 2024 patients) revealed a per-patient sensitivity of 96%, specificity of 74%, and positive and negative predictive values of 68% and 97%, respectively.[45] Two prospective multicenter studies reporting the accuracy of CCTA have been published recently.[46,47] In patients with no known CAD the criterion for enrollment in the Assessment by Coronary Computed Tomographic Angiography of Individuals Undergoing Invasive Coronary Angiography [ACCURACY] trial, the sensitivity, specificity, positive predictive value, and negative predictive value were 95%, 83%, 64%, and 99%, respectively.[46] Conversely, 20% of patients in the Coronary Evaluation using Multislice Spiral CTA using 64 Detectors (CORE 64) trial had known CAD resulting in sensitivity, specificity, positive predictive, and negative predictive values of 85%, 90%, 91%, and 83%, respectively.[47] As expected, the diagnostic performance of CCTA depends somewhat on the prevalence of CAD. A comprehensive review of the diagnostic accuracy of CCTA is provided in the article by Thompson elsewhere in this issue.

The comparative capability of CCTA for quantitative analysis of coronary lesion severity has also been studied.[8,24,25] Generally, good correlation values with invasive angiography are found (average Pearson correlation, $r$ = 0.72) but with considerable standard deviation, which presently limits its quantitative accuracy. The severity of lesions on CCTA does not directly translate into stenosis grade on invasive angiography because CCTA has much greater flexibility in assessing lesions from multiple viewing angles, with the extent of disease in diffusely diseased segments being easily discerned.

## CORONARY CT ANGIOGRAPHY IN THE EMERGENCY DEPARTMENT

In patients with a low to intermediate probability of CAD (eg, those presenting to the ED), CCTA performs well in ruling out CAD, and American College of Cardiology (ACC) and American Heart Association (AHA) guidelines deem this application to be "appropriate".[48,49] In patients with a high pretest probability, CCTA may not provide additional relevant diagnostic information.[48]

A randomized controlled study was performed at the authors' center to evaluate the use of CCTA versus standard of care in 200 low- to intermediate-risk patients with acute chest pain.[50] Patients randomized to immediate CCTA were eligible for discharge with normal or minimally abnormal results (<25% stenosis), and patients with severe stenosis (>70%) were referred for immediate invasive angiography, whereas patients with intermediate-grade stenoses underwent stress testing. In the standard-of-care arm, patients were eligible for discharge if the results of serial ECG scans and cardiac enzyme levels were negative and stress-testing results were normal, whereas those with abnormal stress test results were referred for cardiac catheterization. The two groups were compared for safety, diagnostic accuracy, and efficiency. Minimal or no CAD was demonstrated in 67% of the CCTA group, resulting in rapid discharge of these patients from the ED with a diagnosis of noncoronary chest pain. Among the remainder, 8% had severe stenosis on CCTA prompting immediate admission for invasive angiography. Thus, 75% of patients in the CCTA arm underwent prompt triage based on CCTA findings, resulting in reduction of diagnostic time by 77%, (ie, 3.4 hours compared with 15 hours in the standard-of-care arm). Importantly, CCTA was found to be safe, with no test complications or a subsequent diagnosis of CAD or major adverse cardiac events over the next 6 months. Overall, the diagnostic accuracy of CCTA was 94%, with a negative predictive value of 100%, similar to a recent pooled analysis of six studies in 445 patients (overall sensitivity, specificity, positive predictive, and negative predictive values to detect ACS were 95%, 86%, 61%, and 99%, respectively).[51] The Coronary Computed Tomography for Systematic Triage of Acute Chest Pain Patients to Treatment (CT-STAT) trial with an identical study design involving 750 patients at 15 centers across the United States has recently completed enrollment; this study has the potential to provide a further evidence base for the clinical use of CCTA in the ED.

In addition to the expedited triage of patients with chest pain in the ED (**Fig. 1**), an important

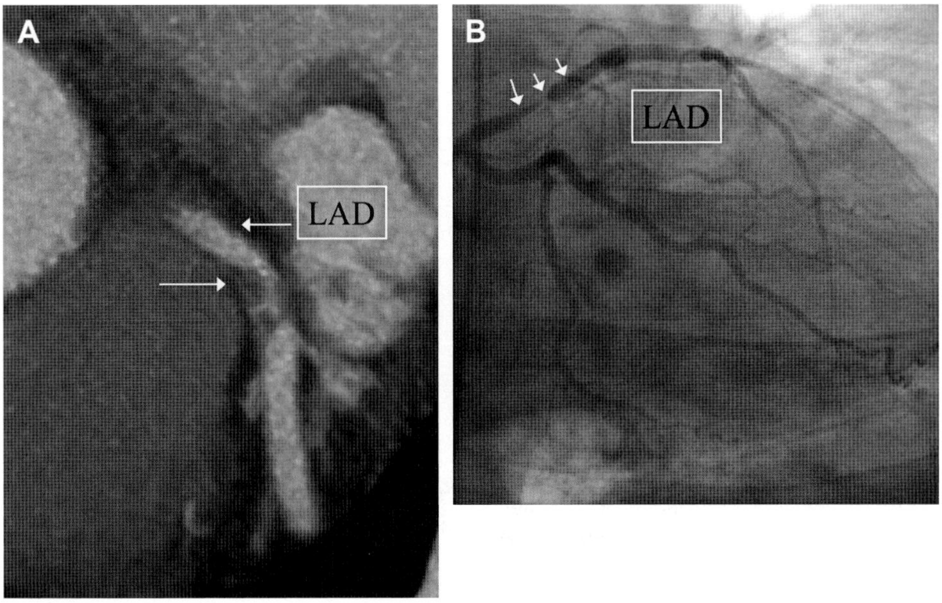


**Fig. 1.** (*A*) CCTA of a 55-year-old man who presented to the emergency center with stuttering chest pain. The ECG scan was unremarkable, and cardiac enzymes were negative. High-grade noncalcified plaque is visualized in the proximal left anterior descending (LAD) artery (*arrows*). (*B*) Patient underwent urgent invasive coronary angiography with percutaneous revascularization of the LAD (*arrows*) with excellent angiographic results.

consideration for use of this technology is the decrease in absolute costs. In the authors' study, this approach resulted in a decrease in cost by 16% ($1586 in the CCTA arm compared with $1872 in the standard-of-care arm).[50] In a study by Rubinshtein and colleagues,[52] the need for hospitalization among patients with acute chest pain was shown to decrease by nearly 50% with a CCTA-based approach.

### *Noncardiac Causes of Chest Pain: The "Triple Rule-Out" Protocol and Beyond*

In the process of acquiring CCTA images, three-dimensional data are acquired from the entire thorax within the field of view. This routine acquisition results in the ability to examine other noncardiac structures, such as the aorta and pulmonary arteries, providing an attractive modality for ruling out the three most potentially fatal causes of chest pain: CAD, acute aortic dissection, and pulmonary embolism (**Fig. 2**). The major technical challenge of a triple rule-out scan protocol is to obtain high and consistent contrast intensity in all three vascular beds, mandating a carefully tailored imaging and injection protocol. In one study, a triphasic injection protocol and caudal-cranial scan acquisition resulted in consistently good opacification (>250 Hounsfield units) of the mean coronary artery, pulmonary artery, and aorta.[53] Compared with the 10- and 16-slice protocols specifically timed for the aorta or the pulmonary arteries, a triphasic protocol results in higher attenuation values in all three vascular beds.[54]

Nearly one in six patients without CAD detected on CCTA has noncardiac findings that could explain the presenting symptoms.[55] Although the "triple rule-out" protocol can diagnose a myriad of cardiac and noncardiac pathologic findings, it should not be used unless there is a high index of suspicion for two of the three pathologic findings in question, because prior studies of patients with acute chest pain have shown that the incidence of occult pulmonary embolism or aortic dissection in patients without suggestive signs or symptoms is low.[56] Additionally, radiation dose is directly proportional to the scan length, increasing by 30% to 50% in triple rule-out scans.

In most centers, noncoronary cardiac images and noncardiac thoracic images are examined on a routine basis and major structures, such as the great vessels, cardiac chambers, valves, and pericardial structures, are defined at high resolution.[57] Multiplanar images can be created at specific increments (eg, every 10%) throughout the R-R interval to form short-axis cine images of the left ventricle from base to apex for evaluation of left ventricular function.

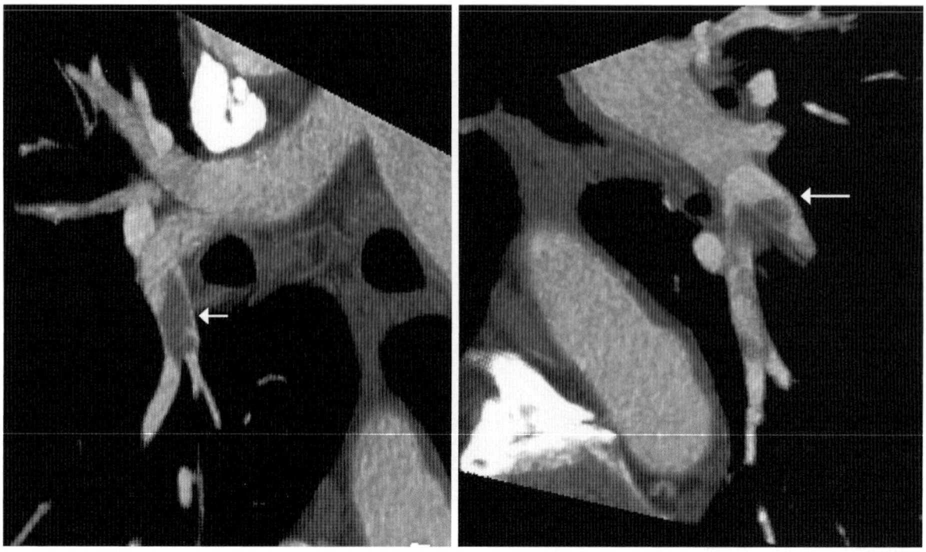

Fig. 2. Triple rule-out protocol was used in a 67-year old man presenting with chest pain, severe epigastric pain, and dyspnea with negative cardiac enzymes and no acute ECG changes. He was found to have bilateral lower lobe pulmonary emboli (*arrow*). The coronary anatomy was unremarkable.

## LIMITATIONS OF CORONARY CT ANGIOGRAPHY

CCTA has several important limitations that affect its usefulness in the triage of patients with acute chest pain in the ED. Although development of 64-slice spiral CT systems was accompanied by an increase in gantry rotation speed (330 milliseconds) and improved temporal resolution (temporal resolution of 165 milliseconds with half-scan reconstruction), the scanning algorithms of these systems display a nonlinear relation to heart rate, making them sensitive to changes in heart rate during image acquisition.[58] Even with the new-generation 64-slice CT scanners, image quality is inversely correlated to heart rate, requiring premedication with beta-blockers to lower heart rates during acquisition in most patients. Nearly 15% of patients in the ED have some contraindication to beta-blockers, rendering them unsuitable for CCTA.[56] If available, dual-source or other novel scanners may obviate the need for beta-blocker administration in most such patients. In addition, because ECG-gating is critical to coronary imaging, any arrhythmias, ectopy, or ECG artifacts result in degradation of image quality. Currently, CCTA in atrial fibrillation is a more difficult examination and requires specialized acquisition and reconstruction protocols. New scanner improvements may make acquisition possible within a single heartbeat, making high-quality results during arrhythmias consistently available.

Extensive coronary calcification obscures the lumen and may substantially limit analysis of segments or even entire arteries by CCTA. Thus, this technique may be of limited application in patients with a high likelihood of significant coronary calcification, such as the elderly, or in patients with prior calcium scores greater than 1000 Agatston units.[23,31,59] Similarly, patients with preexisting CAD often have extensive coronary calcifications, known intermediate-severity coronary lesions; coronary stents with resultant metal artifacts; or prior coronary bypass grafting with extensively calcified native vessels and small-caliber distal coronary arteries. Consideration should be given to the relative risk for any patient with acute chest pain who has a calcium score of 400 or greater even if discrete stenoses cannot be identified. Additionally, in most patients, known prior coronary disease implies that many lesions may be revealed by CCTA; the question is not whether CAD is present but whether it is causing ischemia, which is better answered by physiologic testing than anatomic testing.

Obesity increases radiation scatter within the patient's body and, consequently, degrades image quality as the result of a reduction in the signal-to-noise ratio. All these factors diminish the diagnostic accuracy of CCTA, rendering it probably inappropriate for ED triage in patients with a body mass index greater than 35 kg/m$^2$. Again, technical advances exist on dual-source scanners that have extended the capability of CCTA to image morbidly obese patients with good image quality.[60]

Radiation exposure is a significant consideration in CCTA, resulting in a nonnegligible lifetime attributable risk for cancer, and this should be weighed against potential benefits, especially in sensitive populations, such as women younger than 45 years of age.[61] In a recently published survey of 1965 CCTA examinations at 50 study sites, Hausleiter and colleagues[62] reported a median dose of 12 mSv. Importantly, a wide variation was noted in the median dose between sites and scanner systems, and dose reduction techniques were not uniformly used. This figure is similar to doses reported from myocardial perfusion scans using technetium and less than that of scans using thallium isotopes.

Dose reduction techniques and avoidance of technical errors is of paramount importance. Radiation dose can be modified by adjusting the tube voltage, tube current, pitch, and scan time. Although scan data are acquired and available for the entire phase of the cardiac cycle with retrospective gating, scan data used for image reconstruction are selected only during the diastolic phase. Thus, a high tube current is required only during the diastolic phase (40%–80% of the R-R interval), and a low tube current (decrease by 80%–95%) is acceptable during the remaining cardiac phase ("dose modulation"). This approach of modulating the tube current online with prospective ECG control helps to reduce radiation exposure substantially (up to 47% depending on heart rate) without decreasing diagnostic image quality.[63]

Further reduction in radiation dose can be accomplished by using a lower tube voltage (eg, 100 kV in nonobese patients).[64] Some groups have recently investigated the use of "prospective" gating only (in which data are acquired for a short segment in diastole only) for patients with a low and stable heart rate, yielding total radiation doses less than 5 mSv, with no compromise in image quality compared with retrospective gating.[65,66]

An important consideration is that CCTA, just as with invasive angiography, delineates anatomy only, and can therefore only infer the impact of any given luminal narrowing on coronary blood flow. Anatomic assessment of the coronaries is most clinically reassuring when the vessels are normal or have minimal disease and may reliably predict the physiologic significance of severe stenoses. Anatomic data, by themselves, are limited in assessing the physiologic significance of stenoses of "intermediate severity" (30%–70% diameter stenoses), however. Whether such anatomically defined lesions are responsible for symptoms or are "innocent bystanders" requires adjudication by physiologic determination of coronary blood flow.[67]

## RECOMMENDATION FOR A CORONARY CT ANGIOGRAPHY–BASED EMERGENCY DEPARTMENT TRIAGE PROTOCOL

A team approach is required to implement a CCTA-based ED triage protocol. ED physicians and expert CCTA interpreters must be well educated regarding the application and inherent limitations of CCTA. Patient selection must be rigorous to avoid the potential for overuse of CCTA and to avoid unnecessary radiation.

CCTA is not recommended in patients with a high-risk profile (positive cardiac enzymes or acute ECG changes). Such patients must be managed according to the standard of care at their local institution in accordance with the ACC and AHA guidelines (**Fig. 3**). Additionally, CCTA is generally not recommended in patients with acute chest pain and a known history of CAD, including prior coronary artery bypass grafting surgery or coronary stents. Although the reported accuracy for detection of in-stent restenosis is good (sensitivity and specificity of 86% and 98%, respectively, in one study),[68] adequate stent visualization heavily depends on stent size and material and on modification of image acquisition and reconstruction protocols.[69,70]

Similarly, although CCTA is an excellent tool for evaluation of bypass graft stenosis and patency with sensitivity and specificity in the 90% to 95% range,[71–73] the native coronary arteries of such patients are often so heavily calcified and diffusely diseased that assessment of the run-off vessels is incomplete. This may not be desirable in patients with acute chest pain when identification of the culprit is particularly important. In patients with known CAD and a non–high-risk profile, a stress test–based approach is recommended.

## FUTURE DIRECTIONS

Atherosclerosis of the coronary arteries is a dynamic process, with stable disease interspersed with periods of instability and rapid increase in plaque volume.[74,75] Additionally, most AMIs result from atherosclerotic plaques previously demonstrating less than 50% stenosis on angiography.[76] Invasive angiographic studies have demonstrated the role of the vulnerable plaque and its rupture in myocardial infarction, even in the absence of significant luminal stenosis. Vulnerable plaques are associated with a thin fibrous cap, large lipid core, and inflammatory cells.[77–79] Characterization of plaque, in addition to severity, particularly in patients with chest pain, may be important. One study examining patients presenting with ACS reported plaque

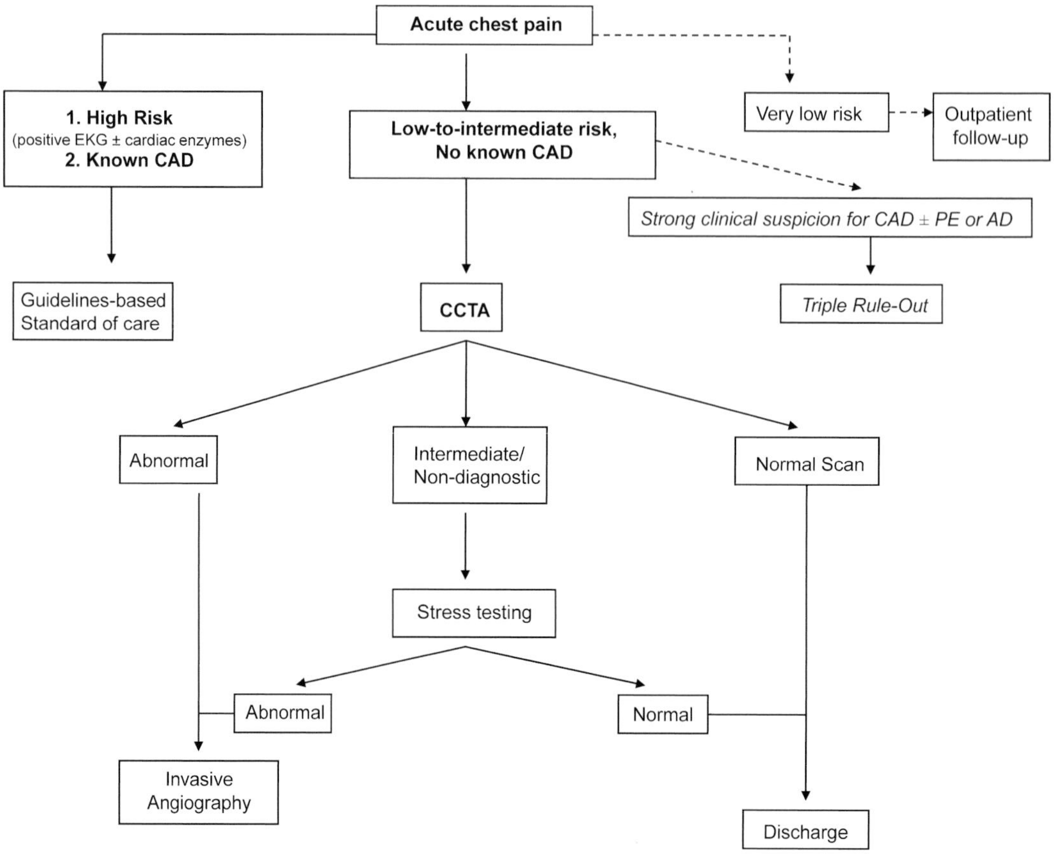


**Fig. 3.** Suggested algorithm for a CCTA-based protocol in evaluation of patients with acute chest pain in the emergency department. PE, pulmonary embolism; AD, acute aortic dissection.

morphology similar to that seen on invasive angiography, with characteristics of plaque disruption, including lesion haziness, positive remodeling, ulceration, and intraplaque contrast penetration.[80] Hoffmann and colleagues[81] have demonstrated a higher plaque burden and remodeling in patients with ACS compared with those with stable angina. Currently, however, plaque characterization is limited to images of extremely high quality and may not be applicable in average clinical practice.[82–84]

Cardiac CT also has potential for evaluation of myocardial perfusion and viability. Quantitative analysis of myocardial perfusion is based primarily on differences in CT attenuation values and the ability to assess areas of myocardial hypoattenuation adequately, which is indicative of diminished myocardial perfusion.[85] This application can be of use in patients with chest pain in the ED and in lesions of intermediate severity, with the possibility of a "one-stop shop."

Historically, ED evaluation of patients with acute chest pain has entailed lengthy and expensive diagnostic testing. Preliminary research suggests that the application of CCTA can potentially revolutionize the evaluation of appropriately selected patients. Multicenter trials are in progress to determine if these promising single-center studies can be confirmed. Also, continuing research is ongoing into novel diagnostic strategies, including CT myocardial perfusion imaging and evaluation of plaque morphology, that may expedite further the care of this large patient population. Although the future of this technology holds great promise, the limitations and risks, particularly that of radiation exposure, must be considered carefully before selection of patients for CCTA.

## REFERENCES

1. McCaig LF, Burt CW. The National Hospital Ambulatory Medical Care Survey: 2003 emergency department summary. In: CDC. National Center for Health Statistics, Centers for Disease Control and Prevention. Advance data from vital and health statistics. Hyattsville: Maryland: CDC; 2005. p. 358.

2. Kohn MA, Kwan E, Gupta M, et al. Prevalence of acute myocardial infarction and other serious diagnoses in patients presenting to an urban emergency department with chest pain. J Emerg Med 2005;29:383–90.
3. Lee TH, Rouan GW, Weisberg MC, et al. Clinical characteristics and natural history of patients with acute myocardial infarction sent home from the emergency room. Am J Cardiol 1987;60:219–24.
4. Pope JH, Aufderheide TP, Ruthazer R, et al. Missed diagnoses of acute cardiac ischemia in the emergency department. N Engl J Med 2000;342:1163–70.
5. Lee TH, Goldman L. Evaluation of the patient with acute chest pain. N Engl J Med 2000;342:1187–95.
6. Braunwald E, Antman EM, Beasley JW, et al. ACC/AHA 2002 guideline update for the management of patients with unstable angina and non-ST-segment elevation myocardial infarction—summary article: a report of the American College of Cardiology/American Heart Association Task Force on Practice Guidelines (Committee on the Management of Patients with Unstable Angina). J Am Coll Cardiol 2002;40:1366–74.
7. Hamm CW, Goldmann BU, Heeschen C, et al. Emergency room triage of patients with acute chest pain by means of rapid testing for cardiac troponin T or troponin I. N Engl J Med 1997;337:1648–53.
8. Meinertz T, Hamm CW. Rapid testing for cardiac troponins in patients with acute chest pain in the emergency room. Eur Heart J 1998;19:973–4.
9. Singer AJ, Ardise J, Gulla J, et al. Point-of-care testing reduces length of stay in emergency department chest pain patients. Ann Emerg Med 2005;45:587–91.
10. Svensson L, Axelsson C, Nordlander R, et al. Prognostic value of biochemical markers, 12-lead ECG and patient characteristics amongst patients calling for an ambulance due to a suspected acute coronary syndrome. J Intern Med 2004;255:469–77.
11. Tatum JL, Jesse RL, Kontos MC, et al. Comprehensive strategy for the evaluation and triage of the chest pain patient. Ann Emerg Med 1997;29:116–25.
12. Heller GV, Stowers SA, Hendel RC, et al. Clinical value of acute rest technetium-99m tetrofosmin tomographic myocardial perfusion imaging in patients with acute chest pain and nondiagnostic electrocardiograms. J Am Coll Cardiol 1998;31:1011–7.
13. Sicari R, Pasanisi E, Venneri L, et al. Stress echo results predict mortality: a large-scale multicenter prospective international study. J Am Coll Cardiol 2003;41:589–95.
14. Wackers FJ, Brown KA, Heller GV, et al. American Society of Nuclear Cardiology position statement on radionuclide imaging in patients with suspected acute ischemic syndromes in the emergency department or chest pain center. J Nucl Cardiol 2002;9:246–50.
15. Jeudy J, White CS. Evaluation of acute chest pain in the emergency department: utility of multidetector computed tomography. Semin Ultrasound CT MR 2007;28:109–14.
16. Motoyama S, Anno H, Sarai M, et al. Noninvasive coronary angiography with a prototype 256-row area detector computed tomography system: comparison with conventional invasive coronary angiography. J Am Coll Cardiol 2008;51:773–5.
17. Rybicki FJ, Otero HJ, Steigner ML, et al. Initial evaluation of coronary images from 320-detector row computed tomography. Int J Cardiovasc Imaging 2008;24:535–46.
18. Achenbach S, Ropers D, Pohle FK, et al. Detection of coronary artery stenoses using multi-detector CT with 16 × 0.75 collimation and 375 ms rotation. Eur Heart J 2005;26:1978–86.
19. Caussin C, Daoud B, Ghostine S, et al. Comparison of lumens of intermediate coronary stenosis using 16-slice computed tomography versus intravascular ultrasound. Am J Cardiol 2005;96:524–8.
20. Fine JJ, Hopkins CB, Ruff N, et al. Comparison of accuracy of 64-slice cardiovascular computed tomography with coronary angiography in patients with suspected coronary artery disease. Am J Cardiol 2006;97:173–4.
21. Garcia MJ, Lessick J, Hoffmann MH. Accuracy of 16-row multidetector computed tomography for the assessment of coronary artery stenosis. JAMA 2006;296:403–11.
22. Ghostine S, Caussin C, Daoud B, et al. Non-invasive detection of coronary artery disease in patients with left bundle branch block using 64-slice computed tomography. J Am Coll Cardiol 2006;48:1929–34.
23. Gilard M, Cornily JC, Pennec PY, et al. Accuracy of multislice computed tomography in the preoperative assessment of coronary disease in patients with aortic valve stenosis. J Am Coll Cardiol 2006;47:2020–4.
24. Hoffmann MH, Shi H, Schmitz BL, et al. Noninvasive coronary angiography with multislice computed tomography. JAMA 2005;293:2471–8.
25. Kefer J, Coche E, Legros G, et al. Head-to-head comparison of three-dimensional navigator-gated magnetic resonance imaging and 16-slice computed tomography to detect coronary artery stenosis in patients. J Am Coll Cardiol 2005;46:92–100.
26. Kuettner A, Beck T, Drosch T, et al. Diagnostic accuracy of noninvasive coronary imaging using 16-detector slice spiral computed tomography with 188 ms temporal resolution. J Am Coll Cardiol 2005;45:123–7.
27. Kuettner A, Trabold T, Schroeder S, et al. Noninvasive detection of coronary lesions using 16-detector

multislice spiral computed tomography technology: initial clinical results. J Am Coll Cardiol 2004;44: 1230–7.
28. Leber AW, Knez A, von Ziegler F, et al. Quantification of obstructive and nonobstructive coronary lesions by 64-slice computed tomography: a comparative study with quantitative coronary angiography and intravascular ultrasound. J Am Coll Cardiol 2005; 46:147–54.
29. Leschka S, Alkadhi H, Plass A, et al. Accuracy of MSCT coronary angiography with 64-slice technology: first experience. Eur Heart J 2005;26: 1482–7.
30. Lim MC, Wong TW, Yaneza LO, et al. Noninvasive detection of significant coronary artery disease with multi-section computed tomography angiography in patients with suspected coronary artery disease. Clin Radiol 2006;61:174–80.
31. Manghat NE, Morgan-Hughes GJ, Broadley AJ, et al. 16-Detector row computed tomographic coronary angiography in patients undergoing evaluation for aortic valve replacement: comparison with catheter angiography. Clin Radiol 2006;61:749–57.
32. Martuscelli E, Romagnoli A, D'Eliseo A, et al. Accuracy of thin-slice computed tomography in the detection of coronary stenoses. Eur Heart J 2004;25:1043–8.
33. Meijboom WB, Mollet NR, Van Mieghem CA, et al. Pre-operative computed tomography coronary angiography to detect significant coronary artery disease in patients referred for cardiac valve surgery. J Am Coll Cardiol 2006;48:1658–65.
34. Mollet NR, Cademartiri F, Krestin GP, et al. Improved diagnostic accuracy with 16-row multi-slice computed tomography coronary angiography. J Am Coll Cardiol 2005;45:128–32.
35. Mollet NR, Cademartiri F, Nieman K, et al. Multislice spiral computed tomography coronary angiography in patients with stable angina pectoris. J Am Coll Cardiol 2004;43:2265–70.
36. Mollet NR, Cademartiri F, Nieman K, et al. Noninvasive assessment of coronary plaque burden using multislice computed tomography. Am J Cardiol 2005;95:1165–9.
37. Mollet NR, Cademartiri F, van Mieghem CA, et al. High-resolution spiral computed tomography coronary angiography in patients referred for diagnostic conventional coronary angiography. Circulation 2005;112:2318–23.
38. Morgan-Hughes GJ, Marshall AJ, Roobottom CA. Multislice computed tomographic coronary angiography: experience in a UK centre. Clin Radiol 2003;58:378–83.
39. Nieman K, Oudkerk M, Rensing BJ, et al. Coronary angiography with multi-slice computed tomography. Lancet 2001;357:599–603.
40. Pugliese F, Mollet NR, Runza G, et al. Diagnostic accuracy of non-invasive 64-slice CT coronary angiography in patients with stable angina pectoris. Eur Radiol 2006;16:575–82.
41. Raff GL, Gallagher MJ, O'Neill WW, et al. Diagnostic accuracy of noninvasive coronary angiography using 64-slice spiral computed tomography. J Am Coll Cardiol 2005;46:552–7.
42. Reant P, Brunot S, Lafitte S, et al. Predictive value of noninvasive coronary angiography with multidetector computed tomography to detect significant coronary stenosis before valve surgery. Am J Cardiol 2006;97:1506–10.
43. Ropers D, Baum U, Pohle K, et al. Detection of coronary artery stenoses with thin-slice multi-detector row spiral computed tomography and multiplanar reconstruction. Circulation 2003;107:664–6.
44. Ropers D, Rixe J, Anders K, et al. Usefulness of multidetector row spiral computed tomography with 64- × 0.6-mm collimation and 330-ms rotation for the noninvasive detection of significant coronary artery stenoses. Am J Cardiol 2006;97:343–8.
45. Hamon M, Biondi-Zoccai GG, Malagutti P, et al. Diagnostic performance of multislice spiral computed tomography of coronary arteries as compared with conventional invasive coronary angiography: a meta-analysis. J Am Coll Cardiol 2006; 48:1896–910.
46. Budoff MJ, Dowe D, Jollis JG, et al. Diagnostic performance of 64-multidetector row coronary computed tomographic angiography for evaluation of coronary artery stenosis in individuals without known coronary artery disease: results from the prospective multicenter ACCURACY (Assessment by Coronary Computed Tomographic Angiography of Individuals Undergoing Invasive Coronary Angiography) trial. J Am Coll Cardiol 2008;52:1724–32.
47. Miller JM, Rochitte CE, Dewey M, et al. Diagnostic performance of coronary angiography by 64-row CT. N Engl J Med 2008;359:2324–36.
48. Meijboom WB, van Mieghem CA, Mollet NR, et al. 64-Slice computed tomography coronary angiography in patients with high, intermediate, or low pretest probability of significant coronary artery disease. J Am Coll Cardiol 2007;50:1469–75.
49. Hendel RC, Patel MR, Kramer CM, et al. ACCF/ACR/SCCT/SCMR/ASNC/NASCI/SCAI/SIR 2006 appropriateness criteria for cardiac computed tomography and cardiac magnetic resonance imaging: a report of the American College of Cardiology Foundation Quality Strategic Directions Committee Appropriateness Criteria Working Group, American College of Radiology, Society of Cardiovascular Computed Tomography, Society for Cardiovascular Magnetic Resonance, American Society of Nuclear Cardiology, North American Society for Cardiac Imaging, Society for Cardiovascular Angiography and Interventions, and Society of Interventional Radiology. J Am Coll Cardiol 2006;48:1475–97.

50. Goldstein JA, Gallagher MJ, O'Neill WW, et al. A randomized controlled trial of multi-slice coronary computed tomography for evaluation of acute chest pain. J Am Coll Cardiol 2007;49:863–71.
51. Cury RC, Feutchner G, Pena CS, et al. Acute chest pain imaging in the emergency department with cardiac computed tomography angiography. J Nucl Cardiol 2008;15:564–75.
52. Rubinshtein R, Halon DA, Gaspar T, et al. Impact of 64-slice cardiac computed tomographic angiography on clinical decision-making in emergency department patients with chest pain of possible myocardial ischemic origin. Am J Cardiol 2007; 100:1522–6.
53. Vrachliotis TG, Bis KG, Haidary A, et al. Atypical chest pain: coronary, aortic, and pulmonary vasculature enhancement at biphasic single-injection 64-section CT angiography. Radiology 2007;243: 368–76.
54. Haidary A, Bis K, Vrachliotis T, et al. Enhancement performance of a 64-slice triple rule-out protocol versus 16-slice and 10-slice multidetector CT-angiography protocols for evaluation of aortic and pulmonary vasculature. J Comput Assist Tomogr 2007;31:917–23.
55. Onuma Y, Tanabe K, Nakazawa G, et al. Noncardiac findings in cardiac imaging with multidetector computed tomography. J Am Coll Cardiol 2006;48: 402–6.
56. Gallagher MJ, Raff GL. Use of multislice CT for the evaluation of emergency room patients with chest pain: the so-called "triple rule-out". Catheter Cardiovasc Interv 2008;71:92–9.
57. Woodard PK, Bhalla S, Javidan-Nejad C, et al. Noncoronary cardiac CT imaging. Semin Ultrasound CT MR 2006;27:56–75.
58. Achenbach S, Ropers D, Kuettner A, et al. Contrast-enhanced coronary artery visualization by dual-source computed tomography—initial experience. Eur J Radiol 2006;57:331–5.
59. Agatston AS, Janowitz WR, Hildner FJ, et al. Quantification of coronary artery calcium using ultrafast computed tomography. J Am Coll Cardiol 1990;15: 827–32.
60. Chinnaiyan KM, McCullough PA, Flohr TG, et al. Improved noninvasive coronary angiography in morbidly obese patients with dual-source computed tomography. J Cardiovasc Comput Tomogr 2008; 3(1):35–42.
61. Einstein AJ, Henzlova MJ, Rajagopalan S. Estimating risk of cancer associated with radiation exposure from 64-slice computed tomography coronary angiography. JAMA 2007;298:317–23.
62. Hausleiter J, Meyer T, Hermann F, et al. Estimated radiation dose associated with cardiac CT angiography. JAMA 2009;301:500–7.
63. Morin RL, Gerber TC, McCollough CH. Radiation dose in computed tomography of the heart. Circulation 2003;107:917–22.
64. Chinnaiyan KM, McCullough PA. Optimizing outcomes in coronary CT imaging. Rev Cardiovasc Med 2008;9:215–24.
65. Husmann L, Valenta I, Gaemperli O, et al. Feasibility of low-dose coronary CT angiography: first experience with prospective ECG-gating. Eur Heart J 2008;29:191–7.
66. Shuman WP, Branch KR, May JM, et al. Prospective versus retrospective ECG gating for 64-detector CT of the coronary arteries: comparison of image quality and patient radiation dose. Radiology 2008; 248:431–7.
67. Goldstein J, et al. CT angiography to deduce coronary physiology. Cathet Cardiovasc Interv 2009; 73(4):503–5.
68. Schuijf JD, Bax JJ, Jukema JW, et al. Feasibility of assessment of coronary stent patency using 16-slice computed tomography. Am J Cardiol 2004;94:427–30.
69. Maintz D, Seifarth H, Flohr T, et al. Improved coronary artery stent visualization and in-stent stenosis detection using 16-slice computed-tomography and dedicated image reconstruction technique. Invest Radiol 2003;38:790–5.
70. Rixe J, Achenbach S, Ropers D, et al. Assessment of coronary artery stent restenosis by 64-slice multi-detector computed tomography. Eur Heart J 2006; 27:2567–72.
71. Gilkeson RC, Markowitz AH. Multislice CT evaluation of coronary artery bypass graft patients. J Thorac Imaging 2007;22:56–62.
72. Pache G, Saueressig U, Frydrychowicz A, et al. Initial experience with 64-slice cardiac CT: non-invasive visualization of coronary artery bypass grafts. Eur Heart J 2006;27:976–80.
73. Schlosser T, Konorza T, Hunold P, et al. Noninvasive visualization of coronary artery bypass grafts using 16-detector row computed tomography. J Am Coll Cardiol 2004;44:1224–9.
74. Kher N, Marsh JD. Pathobiology of atherosclerosis—a brief review. Semin Thromb Hemost 2004;30: 665–72.
75. Libby P, Ridker PM. Inflammation and atherothrombosis: from population biology and bench research to clinical practice. J Am Coll Cardiol 2006;48:33–46.
76. Little WC, Constantinescu M, Applegate RJ, et al. Can coronary angiography predict the site of a subsequent myocardial infarction in patients with mild-to-moderate coronary artery disease? Circulation 1988;78:1157–66.
77. Falk E, Shah PK, Fuster V. Coronary plaque disruption. Circulation 1995;92:657–71.
78. Naghavi M, Libby P, Falk E, et al. From vulnerable plaque to vulnerable patient: a call for new

definitions and risk assessment strategies: part I. Circulation 2003;108:1664–72.
79. Stary HC, Chandler AB, Dinsmore RE, et al. A definition of advanced types of atherosclerotic lesions and a histological classification of atherosclerosis. A report from the Committee on Vascular Lesions of the Council on Arteriosclerosis, American Heart Association. Circulation 1995;92:1355–74.
80. Goldstein JA, Dixon SR, Safian RD, et al. Computed tomographic angiographic morphology of invasively proven complex coronary plaques. J Am Coll Cardiol Img 2008;1:249–51.
81. Hoffmann U, Moselewski F, Nieman K, et al. Noninvasive assessment of plaque morphology and composition in culprit and stable lesions in acute coronary syndrome and stable lesions in stable angina by multidetector computed tomography. J Am Coll Cardiol 2006;47:1655–62.
82. Achenbach S, Moselewski F, Ropers D, et al. Detection of calcified and noncalcified coronary atherosclerotic plaque by contrast-enhanced, submillimeter multidetector spiral computed tomography: a segment-based comparison with intravascular ultrasound. Circulation 2004;109:14–7.
83. Bluemke DA, Achenbach S, Budoff M, et al. Noninvasive coronary artery imaging: magnetic resonance angiography and multidetector computed tomography angiography: a scientific statement from the American Heart Association Committee on Cardiovascular Imaging and Intervention of the Council on Cardiovascular Radiology and Intervention, and the Councils on Clinical Cardiology and Cardiovascular Disease in the Young. Circulation 2008;118:586–606.
84. Kim WY, Stuber M, Bornert P, et al. Three-dimensional black-blood cardiac magnetic resonance coronary vessel wall imaging detects positive arterial remodeling in patients with nonsignificant coronary artery disease. Circulation 2002;106:296–9.
85. Cury RC, Nieman K, Shapiro MD, et al. Comprehensive cardiac CT study: evaluation of coronary arteries, left ventricular function, and myocardial perfusion—is it possible? J Nucl Cardiol 2007;14:229–43.

# Functional Versus Anatomic Imaging in Patients with Suspected Coronary Artery Disease

Leslee J. Shaw, PhD, FASNC, FACC[a], Daniel S. Berman, MD[b,*]

KEYWORDS

• Diagnosis • Prognosis • Noninvasive imaging
• CT angiography • Nuclear cardiology

This is an exciting time for the clinical imager, who is availed with an abundance of innovative technologies for advanced imaging of patients with known and suspected coronary artery disease (CAD). Stress myocardial perfusion single-photon emission (SPECT) and positron emission (PET) tomographic myocardial perfusion imaging (MPI) are established techniques that provide information as to the extent and severity of rest- and stress-induced regional myocardial perfusion abnormalities. There is a wealth of available evidence as to the diagnostic and prognostic accuracy of stress MPI that this article discusses. Additionally, a rather recent technique now provides a noninvasive assessment of the location, severity, and extent of anatomic obstructive CAD using coronary computed tomography (CCTA). The burgeoning field of CCTA is evolving rapidly, with recent high-quality evidence as to its diagnostic accuracy from several controlled clinical trials, as well as unfolding evidence as to the prognostic accuracy of this technique.

This article provides a synthesis of available evidence on these two types of noninvasive cardiac imaging: functional evaluation using stress MPI and anatomic evaluation using CCTA. The latter is discussed in terms of its comparative accuracy to magnetic resonance angiography and invasive coronary angiography.

## BASIC PREMISE OF CORRELATING SYMPTOMS WITH IMAGING RISK MARKERS

The main purpose for referral to one of an array of noninvasive imaging procedures is to provide confirmatory correlation between the patient's presenting with signs and symptoms that are suggestive of obstructive CAD and imaging risk markers or abnormalities. Before embarking on a discussion of MPI and CCTA, it is important to realize that there will be a great deal of overlap between these two modalities. That is, patients with high-risk ischemia are also likely to have obstructive CAD. Our understanding of the ischemic cascade can provide us with insight into the potential correlation between MPI abnormalities and obstructive CAD.[1] Coronary atherosclerosis and coronary narrowing often occur without any hemodynamic consequence, and thus would show no abnormality on MPI. When an anatomic stenosis is sufficient to be flow limiting during peak stress, the more severe the defect, the higher the likelihood of a severe coronary stenosis. Severe MPI defects by semiquantitative analysis have been shown to be highly predictive of a critical (>90%) coronary stenosis. However, an MPI abnormality may also be associated with vascular dysfunction in the setting of nonobstructive CAD. In addition, collateral flow in

[a] Emory University School of Medicine, 1256 Briarcliff Rd. NE, Suite 1-N, Atlanta, GA 30306, USA
[b] T-1258 Cedars-Sinai Medical Center, 8700 Beverly Boulevard, Los Angeles, CA 90048, USA
* Corresponding author.
*E-mail address:* daniel.berman@cshs.org (D.S. Berman).

Cardiol Clin 27 (2009) 597–604
doi:10.1016/j.ccl.2009.06.009
0733-8651/09/$ – see front matter 

a patient with obstructive CAD may result in normal flow to that region.[1] It is for this reason that there will be both concordant and discordant findings between MPI and CCTA even when there is no artifact on either examination. Thus, lessons learned from MPI studies on correct identification of an obstructive stenosis include information on the severity of the stenosis, collateral flow, and underlying endothelial function.

This discussion on the relationship between CAD and perfusion ischemia has relevance to the discussion on the comparative accuracy of MPI and CCTA with respect to invasive coronary angiography as a standard. That is, one can expect a fair degree of concordance as to the prevalence of normal studies, as well high-risk studies, which are also likely to be comparable. One exception however, is that a percentage of patients with three-vessel or left-main disease may have balanced reduction in flow that results in underestimation of the extent of perfusion defect by MPI.[1] In contrast, CCTA is highly unlikely to miss high risk CAD. The reported specificity of the two methods is similar. Regarding "normalcy rate", the proxy for specificity once tests are used clinically to determine the need for the gold standard test, MPI and CCTA are similar.[2] Myocardial perfusion PET and, more recently, SPECT imaging can also provide information as to absolute blood flow and coronary flow reserve that may more often detect mild CAD and vascular dysfunction and potentially could be useful in identifying patients with balanced reduction in blood flow that is underestimated by the standard relative perfusion analysis methods. Even without these new measures, there is a fair amount of concordance between individuals with high-risk ischemia and high risk obstructive CAD.

### *Inducible Ischemia with Stress MPI, Obstructive CAD, and Coronary Artery Calcification*

The above discussion is relevant to understanding that although CCTA and MPI are diagnostic procedures, there are reasons for discordant findings. Currently, there are seven reports correlating stress MPI ischemia with CCTA.[3–8] Despite the above premise, the evidence to date notes substantial variability between inducible ischemia and CAD presence and severity that affect diagnostic accuracy and risk detection. Obstructive CAD is often more severe and extensive than the burden of SPECT or PET myocardial ischemia.[5] Moreover, in patients undergoing a test for ischemia and CCTA, less than 25% of patients have concordant abnormal findings.[5] As obstructive CAD prevalence increases, the correlation between stress MPI and angiographic findings improves.[3] For a given lesion with a minimal cross-sectional area less than 3.7 $mm^3$ or stenosis greater than 60%, the sensitivity and specificity of stress MPI is 98% and 84%, respectively.[3] Overall, the postive predictive value for CCTA regarding PET or SPECT ischemia is low; however, this increases as the severity of stenosis increases. An important finding is that the frequency of inducible ischemia has been reported to be 0%, 5%, 33%, 54%, and 86% for CCTA stenosis of 0%, 0% to 60%, 60% to 70%, 70% to 80%, and greater than 80%, respectively ($P$<0001).[3] Another report has shown the accuracy of CCTA for detecting rubidium (Rb) 82 PET ischemia to be 67% for mild CAD (<50% stenosis), 85% for intermediate lesions (50%–70% stenosis), and 93% for significant CAD (>70% stenosis).[9]

As noted above, in some patients, high risk angiographic CAD has been reported to be present in a small proportion of patients with normal MPI.[10] On approach to identifying these patients is to look for ancillary markers on the MPI study such as transient ischemic dilation of the left ventricle, fall in left ventricular ejection fraction, increased lung uptake, and increased right ventricular uptake. Also helpful is taking into account severe clinical responses such as exercise hypotension or severe ST depression. This challenge in detecting multivessel CAD can be handled in part by MPI though considering adding a coronary artery calcification (CAC) study to the MPI examination. This can be accomplished routinely when hybrid PET/CT or SPECT/CT systems are used. Several reports have noted that the addition of CAC to MPI provides incremental value over and above myocardial perfusion findings.[11] That is, for those with normal stress perfusion, adding a CAC score can improve detection of CAD and, importantly, can provide correlative evidence as to a patient's risk of severe or multivessel CAD. It is for this reason that some studies have focused on the addition of CAC to stress MPI in patients with a high likelihood of CAD (eg, diabetics and the elderly).[12] Importantly, adding a CAC scan adds minimal radiation (ie, approximately 1 mSv). For those using combined CAC and MPI, it is noteworthy that evidence of calcified plaque is not site-specific for obstructive CAD,[13] but there is a proportional relationship between CAC extent and inducible ischemia. A statement from the American Society of Nuclear Cardiology synthesizing five reports noted that as the CAC score increased, the frequency of inducible ischemia increased,[14] where ischemia occurs in approximately one in every five patients with a CAC score greater than or equal to 400.[15] A higher frequency of inducible ischemia is expected in diabetic patients, those with the metabolic syndrome, or with a family history of premature CAD and may occur at a lower threshold CAC score greater than or equal to 100.

When integrating findings from CAC and MPI, prognostic estimations for those with a normal MPI will vary depending on the extent of calcification. That is, higher cardiac event rates are reported for patients with normal MPI and high-risk CAC scores.[16,17] For imagers, documentation of high-risk CAC, as a direct marker of atherosclerosis, can help to target patients requiring more intensive risk factor management (perhaps to secondary prevention goals). Finally, it should also be noted that 82Rb PET may also be more accurate than SPECT MPI for the detection of three-vessel or left-main CAD, in particular when adding information on peak stress left-ventricular ejection fraction and wall motion or measurement of coronary flow reserve following stress.[16]

### *Atherosclerotic Plaque and Ischemia*

There are also a few preliminary reports noting that perfusion ischemia occurs more often in the setting of mixed or calcified plaque versus noncalcified plaque.[6,8] These findings put forth intriguing possibilities for improved risk detection using CCTA. Given that mixed or calcified plaques represent a more advanced stage of disease, it makes sense that ischemia would be more prevalent, where constrictive remodeling elicits reductions in myocardial blood flow. Intriguing hypotheses have also been put forth stating that noncalcified plaque is more vulnerable to progression resulting in presentation with an acute coronary syndrome. Thus, documentation of noncalcified plaque may be a harbinger for near-term instability and an associated acute coronary syndrome risk.[18] A report by Motoyama and colleagues[19] revealed that CCTA characteristics of plaque associated with acute coronary syndrome as well as future coronary events in stable patients include constrictive arterial remodeling (ie, coronary stenosis) or low plaque density (ie, noncalcified plaque), as well as spotty calcification, in particular when it surrounds an area of low plaque density (ie, mixed plaque).

## COMPARATIVE DIAGNOSTIC ACCURACY OF STRESS NUCLEAR IMAGING WITH CCTA

There are now three controlled clinical trials on the diagnostic accuracy of 64-slice CCTA compared with invasive coronary angiography, and five meta-analyses on the subject.[20–27] The pooled trial results in 881 patients reveal a diagnostic sensitivity and specificity of 93.8% and 80.2% (**Fig. 1**).[25–27] From a recent meta-analysis, similar accuracy statistics were reported for 64-multislice CCTA with diagnostic sensitivities and specificities of 94% (93%–97%) and 85% (80%–90%).[24] Comparable diagnostic-accuracy results were noted for obese and nonobese patients (a subset for whom MPI may be particularly problematic). The high degree of accuracy and correlation of CCTA with invasive anatomy is expected. One of the strengths of CCTA is its high negative-predictive value, exceeding 95%.[28] The high negative-predictive accuracy could prove advantageous as a diagnostic test for low-intermediate likelihood patients; if CCTA could be performed at a reduced radiation burden of <4 mSv. As expected, a diminished diagnostic specificity was reported for patients with a CAC score greater than 400 and supports the utility of a functional assessment using stress MPI in patients with a high likelihood of extensive CAC (eg, elderly).

### *Diagnostic Accuracy of Stress MPI*

Contemporary MPI has a sensitivity in the range of 85% to 90%.[29] The reported high rate of false-positive (ie, reduced specificity) MPI scans for women and obese patients can be improved with attenuation correction algorithms and incorporation of gated left-ventricular ejection fraction and regional wall motion into the test interpretations, with the result being improved specificity values in the range of 80% to 90%.[30–34] Diagnostic specificity can also be improved by using a prone image to reduce soft tissue-attenuation artifacts.[34] PET imaging has a slightly higher diagnostic sensitivity that is on average 5% to 10% higher than SPECT.[16,35] Importantly, in a recent report using

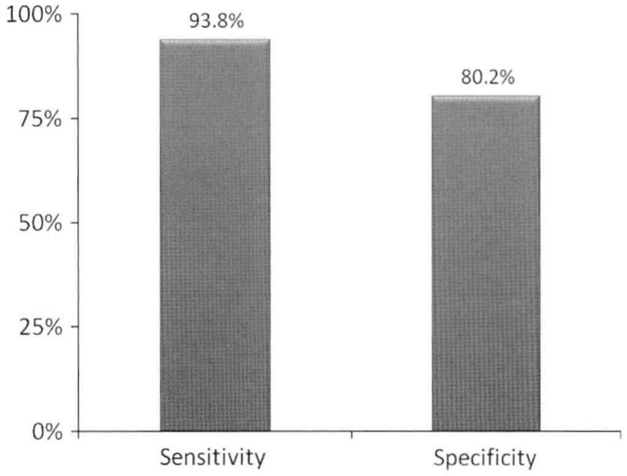


**Fig. 1.** Diagnostic accuracy of 64-slice CCTA in multicenter trials (n = 881 from three trials.) (*Data from* Refs.[24–26]).

82Rb PET-CT, the diagnostic sensitivity was 93%,[36] with detection of multivessel CAD being exceedingly high. As stated above, a major advantage to the use of myocardial perfusion PET is the ability to quantify measures of absolute blood flow and to define areas of dampened coronary flow reserve[37] as well as peak changes in left-ventricular ejection fraction, and the addition of a CAC can further improve its diagnostic accuracy.

Thus, it appears that SPECT MPI has a slightly reduced diagnostic sensitivity when compared to CCTA, but specificity appears similar between the two modalities.

## RISK STRATIFICATION WITH STRESS MPI

There is a wealth of high-quality evidence as to prognostic accuracy for estimation of major adverse cardiovascular events in the near-term (ie, 2–3 years) following abnormal stress MPI,[17] with recent data also in 82Rb PET imaging.[38,39] A synthesis of this finding reveals that as the extent and severity of perfusion abnormalities worsen, the cardiac event rates rise proportionally.

**Fig. 2** plots the cumulative relative risk ratio for CCTA and MPI.[17,40–45] From a meta-analysis, the relative risk for abnormal stress MPI is 6.0 (95% confidence interval or CI, 5.4–7.0).[17]

For patients with normal stress-perfusion results, the annual cardiac death or nonfatal myocardial infarction rate is 0.6%, but varies from a low of 0.3% for women to a high of nearly 2% for patients undergoing pharmacologic stress imaging.[17] Mild MPI abnormalities are associated with higher event rates, generally in the range of 1% to 3%.[40] And, when abnormalities increase to the moderate-severe range, annual event rates are in the 5% to 6% range or even higher, depending on associated risk factors and comorbidity.[46] More recent data are available regarding prognosis with 82Rb PET imaging.[38,39] In a study of 1,441 patients undergoing pharmacologic stress PET, annual mortality rates were 2.4% for a summed stress score (SSS) of 0 to 3, 4.1% for a SSS of 4 to 8, and 6.9% for a SSS of greater

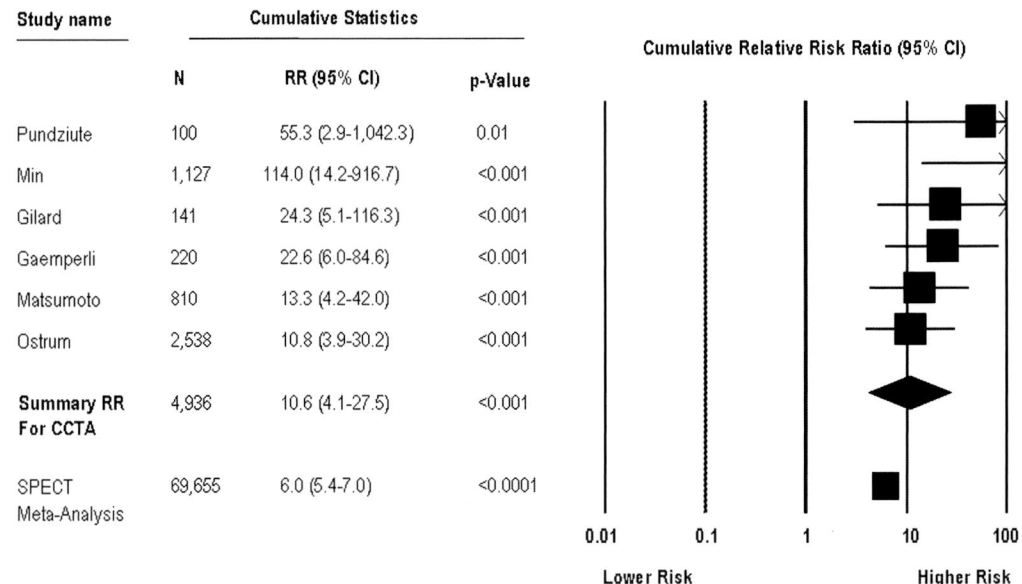

| Study name | Cumulative Statistics | | |
|---|---|---|---|
| | N | RR (95% CI) | p-Value |
| Pundziute | 100 | 55.3 (2.9-1,042.3) | 0.01 |
| Min | 1,127 | 114.0 (14.2-916.7) | <0.001 |
| Gilard | 141 | 24.3 (5.1-116.3) | <0.001 |
| Gaemperli | 220 | 22.6 (6.0-84.6) | <0.001 |
| Matsumoto | 810 | 13.3 (4.2-42.0) | <0.001 |
| Ostrum | 2,538 | 10.8 (3.9-30.2) | <0.001 |
| **Summary RR For CCTA** | 4,936 | 10.6 (4.1-27.5) | <0.001 |
| SPECT Meta-Analysis | 69,655 | 6.0 (5.4-7.0) | <0.0001 |

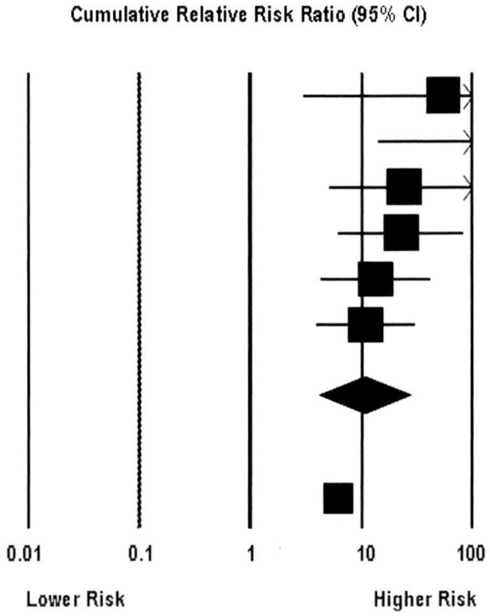


**Fig. 2.** Cumulative relative risk (RR) ratio and 95% confidence intervals (CI) for abnormal or obstructive CAD as compared with no CAD derived from published prognostic series using coronary CT angiography. Over time, the RR have been refined with more narrow CI around the point estimate of 10.6. In a second analysis, the RR for an abnormal versus normal myocardial perfusion SPECT study (as derived from a meta-analysis of Shaw and Iskandrian,[17] and others[40–45]) is also listed for comparative purposes. Although the RR will continue to decline with larger patient series (along with the CI), it appears that the RR is higher for CCTA versus SPECT. Note that a combination of events were used for this calculation, including all-cause mortality, acute myocardial infarction, late revascularization, and unstable angina. Cumulative RR Ratio* was calculated using a Mantel-Haenszel Random Effects Model. To Calculate a RR for Gilard and Matsumoto41, the event data was added solely for no CAD by CCTA. Exclusion of these latter two series does not change the presented results. Note that the heterogeneity statistics for these seven reports was P<.0001. An evaluation of publication bias using this meta-analytic data revealed all but two reports were outside the funnel plot (of the standard error by log odds ratio using random effects calculations).

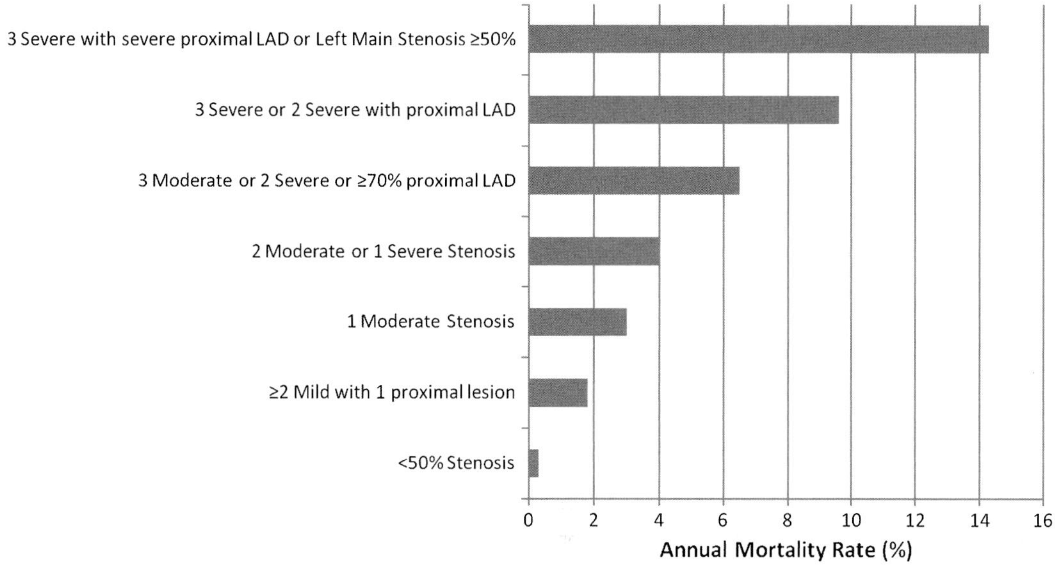


**Fig. 3.** Annual mortality by the Duke CAD Prognostic Index. Stenosis: mild (30%–49%), moderate (50%–69%), and severe (≥70%). *Abbreviation:* LAD, left anterior descending coronary artery. (*Data from* Min JK, Shaw J, Devereux RB, et al. Prognostic value of multidetector coronary computed tomographic angiography for prediction of all-cause mortality. J Am Coll Cardiol 2007;50(12):1161–70.)

than 8, respectively (*P*<.001).[38] In an earlier report of 367 patients, cardiac event rates were 0.4%, 2.3%, and 7.0% per year for normal, mild, and moderate-to-severe stress 82Rb PET findings, respectively.[39] These results are similar to that noted for stress SPECT MPI. It is important to note that 82Rb PET results have been shown to provide improved stratification of risk in obese patients and for those with indeterminate SPECT findings.

## *Prognostic Accuracy of CCTA*

**Fig. 2** also plots the cumulative relative-risk ratio for CCTA evidence of obstructive CAD, as reported from six recent reports in 4,936 patients.[40–45] These results reveal the summary relative-risk ratio for CCTA obstructive CAD is 10.6 (95% CI, 4.1–27.5).[17] Thus, detection of obstructive CAD appears to be associated with a higher risk when compared with identification of stress MPI abnormalities.

From five reports, when the CCTA shows plaque the annual cardiac event rate for patients without obstructive CAD on CCTA was 1.5% (95% CI, 0.9–2.6).[40–45] Thus, it appears that evidence of normal stress MPI may define a lower risk cohort when compared to mild abnormalities on CCTA. Yet, the authors anticipate that additional delineation of risk will unfold as nonobstructive plaque, plaque composition, and arterial remodeling are examined with CCTA such that plaque assessment will refine the prognostic capabilities of the method. Of note, exclusion of any detectable plaque may define the lowest risk cohort of any method–including invasive coronary angiography. Information on this hypothesis has been extensively reported with low-risk CAC scoring where the annual event rate is 0.4%.[13,47]

By comparison, for those with obstructive CAD, the annual cardiac event rate increased to 11.1% (95% CI, 5.1–22.5).[40–45] One would expect that patients with more extensive CAD and those with left-main or proximal left-anterior descending involvement would comprise a subset with even higher clinical outcomes. From one report by Min and colleagues,[41] survival worsened as a function of each increasing category on the Duke CAD Prognostic Index that incorporate stenosis site (proximal) and severity, and the number of obstructive vessels (**Fig. 3**).

## SUMMARY

It is an exciting time in cardiac imaging, where we now have an abundance of high-quality evidence as to the role of stress MPI for diagnosis and risk stratification. Despite its recent entry into the clinical environment, CCTA has rapidly developed extensive diagnostic evidence and rapidly growing prognostic evidence. It appears from a synthesis of this evidence that CCTA has a higher sensitivity for detection of invasively determined obstructive

CAD, as one would expect considering that this is a correlation between two anatomic tests. Clinicians should take care to note the clinical reasons for discordance between a functional and anatomic test. This should also be considered when patients proceed from stress MPI to invasive coronary angiography where nonobstructive CAD is identified. Vascular dysfunction may be present in patients with perfusion abnormalities yet no obstructive CAD. A concerning problem clinically is the finding of normal or mildly abnormal stress MPI in the setting of obstructive CAD. Ancillary findings such as transient ischemic dilation or ejection fraction fall can help identify these high risk patients. A CAC scan may also aid in identifying patients as being at high risk, especially for those with a high likelihood of CAD.

There is a growing body of evidence as to prognosis for CCTA that mirrors the well-established body of evidence with stress MPI. That is, as the extent and severity of CCTA CAD worsens, so do the overall event rates; a similar pattern of directly proportional risk is also noted for stress MPI by the extent and severity of perfusion abnormalities. A recent comparison of annual mortality rates by the percent-ischemic myocardium to a matched cohort undergoing CCTA revealed similar prognostication.[48] It appears for many patients that similar risk-stratification results will be possible for these two modalities. However, one can envision that the exclusion of arterial remodeling and any detectable atherosclerotic plaque may identify a very low-risk patient subset. Moreover, patients with three-vessel or left-main anatomic CAD may also have a higher risk of cardiac events when compared with those with moderate-to-severe perfusion (ie, $\geq$10% myocardium with stress ischemia) abnormalities. Those of us in the field await prospective comparative effectiveness trials or registries so that we can more precisely determine the optimal value of each modality in diverse patient populations as well as to provide evidence regarding the benefit in selected individuals of obtaining both of these examinations.

## REFERENCES


1. Aarnoudse WH, Botman KJ, Pijls NH. False-negative myocardial scintigraphy in balanced three-vessel disease, revealed by coronary pressure measurement. Int J Cardiovasc Intervent 2003;5:67–71.
2. Chow BJW, Abraham A, Wells GA, et al. Diagnostic accuracy and impact of computed tomographic coronary angiography on utilization of invasive coronary angiography. Circ Cardiovasc Imaging 2009;2:16–23.
3. Lin FY, Saba S, Weinsaft JW, et al. Relation of plaque characteristics defined by coronary computed tomographic angiography to ST-segment depression and impaired functional capacity during exercise treadmill testing in patients suspected of having coronary heart disease. Am J Cardiol 2009;103(1):50–8.
4. Sato A, Hiroe M, Tamura M, et al. Quantitative measures of coronary stenosis severity by 64-slice CT angiography and relation to physiologic significance of perfusion in nonobese patients: comparison with stress myocardial perfusion imaging. J Nucl Med 2008;49(4):564–72.
5. Scholte AJ, Schuijf JD, Kharagjitsingh AV, et al. Different manifestations of coronary artery disease by stress SPECT myocardial perfusion imaging, coronary calcium scoring, and multislice CT coronary angiography in asymptomatic patients with type 2 diabetes mellitus. J Nucl Cardiol 2008;15(4):503–9.
6. Esteves FP, Sanyal R, Nye JA, et al. Adenosine stress rubidium-82 PET/computed tomography in patients with known and suspected coronary artery disease. Nucl Med Commun 2008;29(8):674–8.
7. Gaemperli O, Schepis T, Valenta I, et al. Functionally relevant coronary artery disease: comparison of 64-section CT angiography with myocardial perfusion SPECT. Radiology 2008;248(2):414–23.
8. Lin F, Shaw LJ, Berman DS, et al. Multidetector computed tomography coronary artery plaque predictors of stress-induced myocardial ischemia by SPECT. Atherosclerosis 2008;197(2):700–9.
9. Di Carli MF, Dorbala S, Curillova Z, et al. Relationship between CT coronary angiography and stress perfusion imaging in patients with suspected ischemic heart disease assessed by integrated PET-CT imaging. J Nucl Cardiol 2007;14(6):799–809.
10. Berman DS, Kang X, Slomka BJ, et al. Underestimation of extent of ischemia by gated SPECT myocardial perfusion imaging in patients with left main coronary artery disease. J Nucl Cardiol 2007;14:521–8.
11. Schenker MP, Dorbala S, Hong EC, et al. Interrelation of coronary calcification, myocardial ischemia, and outcomes in patients with intermediate likelihood of coronary artery disease: a combined positron emission tomography/computed tomography study. Circulation 2008;117(13):1693–700.
12. Anand DV, Lim E, Hopkins D, et al. Risk stratification in uncomplicated type 2 diabetes: prospective evaluation of the combined use of coronary artery calcium imaging and selective myocardial perfusion scintigraphy. Eur Heart J 2006;27(6):713–21.
13. Greenland P, Bonow RO, Brundage BH, et al. ACCF/AHA 2007 clinical expert consensus document on coronary artery calcium scoring by computed tomography in global cardiovascular risk assessment and in evaluation of patients with chest pain:

a report of the American College of Cardiology Foundation Clinical Expert Consensus Task Force (ACCF/AHA Writing Committee to Update the 2000 Expert Consensus Document on Electron Beam Computed Tomography) developed in collaboration with the Society of Atherosclerosis Imaging and Prevention and the Society of Cardiovascular Computed Tomography. J Am Coll Cardiol 2007; 49(3):378–402.
14. Shaw LJ, Berman DS, Bax JJ, et al. Computed tomography within nuclear cardiology. J Nucl Cardiol 2005; 12:131–42.
15. Berman DS, Wong ND, Gransar H, et al. Relationship between stress-induced myocardial ischemia and atherosclerosis measured by coronary calcium tomography. J Am Coll Cardiol 2004;44(4):923–30.
16. Dorbala S, Vangala D, Sampson U, et al. Value of vasodilator left ventricular ejection fraction reserve in evaluating the magnitude of myocardium at risk and the extent of angiographic coronary artery disease: a 82Rb PET/CT study. J Nucl Med 2007; 48(3):349–58.
17. Shaw LJ, Iskandrian AE. Prognostic value of gated myocardial perfusion SPECT. J Nucl Cardiol 2004; 11(2):171–85.
18. Narula J, Garg P, Achenbach S, et al. Arithmetic of vulnerable plaques for noninvasive imaging. Nat Clin Pract Cardiovasc Med 2008;5(2):S2–10.
19. Motoyama S, Sarai M, Harigaya H, et al. Computed tomographic angiography characteristics of atherosclerotic plaques subsequently resulting in acute coronary syndrome. J Am Coll Cardiol 2009;54: 49–57.
20. Hamon M, Biondi-Zoccai GG, Malagutti P, et al. Diagnostic performance of multislice spiral computed tomography of coronary arteries as compared with conventional invasive coronary angiography: a meta-analysis. J Am Coll Cardiol 2006; 48(9):1896–910.
21. Schuijf JD, Bax JJ, Shaw LJ, et al. Meta-analysis of comparative diagnostic performance of magnetic resonance imaging and multislice computed tomography for noninvasive coronary angiography. Am Heart J 2006;151(2):404–11.
22. Sun Z. Diagnostic accuracy of multislice CT angiography in peripheral arterial disease. J Vasc Interv Radiol 2006;17(12):1915–21.
23. Stein PD, Beemath A, Kayali F, et al. Multidetector computed tomography for the diagnosis of coronary artery disease: a systematic review. Am J Med 2006; 119(3):203–16.
24. Janne d'Othee B, Siebert U, Cury R, et al. A systematic review on diagnostic accuracy of CT-based detection of significant coronary artery disease. Eur J Radiol 2008;65(3):449–61.
25. Budoff MJ, Dowe D, Jollis JG, et al. Diagnostic performance of 64-multidetector row coronary computed tomographic angiography for evaluation of coronary artery stenosis in individuals without known coronary artery disease: results from the prospective multicenter ACCURACY (Assessment by Coronary Computed Tomographic Angiography of Individuals Undergoing Invasive Coronary Angiography) trial. J Am Coll Cardiol 2008;52(21): 1724–32.
26. Miller JM, Rochitte CE, Dewey M, et al. Diagnostic performance of coronary angiography by 64-row CT. N Engl J Med 2008;359(22):2324–36.
27. Meijboom WB, Meijs MF, Schuijf JD, et al. Diagnostic accuracy of 64-slice computed tomography coronary angiography: a prospective, multicenter, multivendor study. J Am Coll Cardiol 2008;52(25):2135–44.
28. Budoff MJ, Achenbach S, Blumenthal RS, et al. Assessment of coronary artery disease by cardiac computed tomography: a scientific statement from the American Heart Association Committee on Cardiovascular Imaging and Intervention, Council on Cardiovascular Radiology and Intervention, and Committee on Cardiac Imaging, Council on Clinical Cardiology. Circulation 2006;114(16):1761–91.
29. Mieres JH, Shaw LJ, Arai A, et al. Role of noninvasive testing in the clinical evaluation of women with suspected coronary artery disease: Consensus statement from the Cardiac Imaging Committee, Council on Clinical Cardiology, and the Cardiovascular Imaging and Intervention Committee, Council on Cardiovascular Radiology and Intervention, American Heart Association. Circulation 2005; 111(5):682–96.
30. Masood Y, Liu YH, Depuey G, et al. Clinical validation of SPECT attenuation correction using x-ray computed tomography-derived attenuation maps: multicenter clinical trial with angiographic correlation. J Nucl Cardiol 2005;12(6):676–86.
31. Fricke E, Fricke H, Weise R, et al. Attenuation correction of myocardial SPECT perfusion images with low-dose CT: evaluation of the method by comparison with perfusion PET. J Nucl Med 2005; 46(5):736–44.
32. Dondi M, Fagioli G, Salgarello M, et al. Myocardial SPECT: what do we gain from attenuation correction (and when)? Q J Nucl Med Mol Imaging 2004;48(3): 181–7.
33. Duvall WL, Croft LB, Corriel JS, et al. SPECT myocardial perfusion imaging in morbidly obese patients: image quality, hemodynamic response to pharmacologic stress, and diagnostic and prognostic value. J Nucl Cardiol 2006;13(2):202–9.
34. Berman DS, Kang X, Nishina H, et al. Diagnostic accuracy of gated Tc-99m Sestamibi stress myocardial perfusion SPECT with combined supine and prone acquisitions to detect coronary artery disease in obese and nonobese patients. J Nucl Cardiol 2006;13(2):191–201.

35. Di Carli MF, Dorbala S, Hachamovitch R. Integrated cardiac PET-CT for the diagnosis and management of CAD. J Nucl Cardiol 2006;13(2):139–44.
36. Sampson UK, Dorbala S, Limaye A, et al. Diagnostic accuracy of rubidium-82 myocardial perfusion imaging with hybrid positron emission tomography/computed tomography in the detection of coronary artery disease. J Am Coll Cardiol 2007;49(10):1052–8.
37. Anagnostopoulos C, Almonacid A, El Fakhri G, et al. Quantitative relationship between coronary vasodilator reserve assessed by 82Rb PET imaging and coronary artery stenosis severity. Eur J Nucl Med Mol Imaging 2008;35(9):1593–601.
38. Lertsburapa K, Ahlberg AW, Bateman TM, et al. Independent and incremental prognostic value of left ventricular ejection fraction determined by stress gated rubidium 82 PET imaging in patients with known or suspected coronary artery disease. J Nucl Cardiol 2008;15(6):745–53.
39. Yoshinaga K, Chow BJ, Williams K, et al. What is the prognostic value of myocardial perfusion imaging using rubidium-82 positron emission tomography? J Am Coll Cardiol 2006;48(5):1029–39.
40. Pundziute G, Schuijf JD, Jukema JW, et al. Prognostic value of multislice computed tomography coronary angiography in patients with known or suspected coronary artery disease. J Am Coll Cardiol 2007;49(1):62–70.
41. Min JK, Shaw LJ, Devereux RB, et al. Prognostic value of multidetector coronary computed tomographic angiography for prediction of all-cause mortality. J Am Coll Cardiol 2007;50(12):1161–70.
42. Gilard M, Le Gal G, Cornily JC, et al. Midterm prognosis of patients with suspected coronary artery disease and normal multislice computed tomographic findings: a prospective management outcome study. Arch Intern Med 2007;167(15):1686–9.
43. Gaemperli O, Valenta I, Schepis T, et al. Coronary 64-slice CT angiography predicts outcome in patients with known or suspected coronary artery disease. Eur Radiol 2008;18(6):1162–73.
44. Matsumoto N, Sato Y, Suzuki Y, et al. Prognostic value of myocardial perfusion single-photon emission computed tomography for the prediction of future cardiac events in a Japanese population: a middle-term follow-up study. Circ J 2007;71(10):1580–5.
45. Ostrom MP, Gopal A, Ahmadi N, et al. Mortality incidence and the severity of coronary atherosclerosis assessed by computed tomography angiography. J Am Coll Cardiol 2008;52(16):1335–43.
46. Berman DS, Kang X, Hayes SW, et al. Adenosine myocardial perfusion single-photon emission computed tomography in women compared with men. Impact of diabetes mellitus on incremental prognostic value and effect on patient management. J Am Coll Cardiol 2003;41(7):1125–33.
47. Bellasi A, Lacey C, Taylor AJ, et al. Comparison of prognostic usefulness of coronary artery calcium in men versus women (results from a meta- and pooled analysis estimating all-cause mortality and coronary heart disease death or myocardial infarction). Am J Cardiol 2007;100(3):409–14.
48. Shaw LJ, Berman DS, Hendel RC, et al. Prognosis by coronary computed tomographic angiography: matched comparison with myocardial perfusion single-photon emission computed tomography. J Cardiovasc Comput Tomogr 2008;2(2):93–101.

# Cardiac CT in Asymptomatic Patients at Risk

Paolo Raggi, MD

**KEYWORDS**

- Atherosclerosis • Coronary calcium
- Computed tomography • Cardiovascular risk

Cardiovascular disease (CVD) is a global health problem, and it is quickly becoming a priority issue even in developing countries. Gender, race, age, genetic, ethnic, and regional variations of risk factors are responsible for the different rates of CVD noted around the world. A look at the published statistics reveals a large disease burden and an associated massive cost. In 2005, the prevalence of CVD in the United States was nearing 81 million people and the associated annual total mortality was almost 870,000 lives. The two most frequent causes of death attributable to CVD were coronary heart disease (52%) and stroke (17%).

## PATHOPHYSIOLOGY OF CORONARY CALCIFICATION

Calcium is a well-known component of the atherosclerotic plaque. Calcification of the atherosclerotic plaque occurs by means of an active process resembling bone formation under the control of complex enzymatic and cellular pathways.[1,2] A large number of in vitro studies have highlighted the involvement of calcium in the process of vascular calcification of osteoblast-like cells, cytokines, transcription factors, and bone morphogenic proteins found in normal bone. Calcification of the intima is characterized by cellular apoptosis,[3] inflammation, lipoprotein, phospholipid accumulation, and, finally, hydroxyapatite deposition. Calcification is first noted in the lipid core of the atheroma, juxtaposed to inflammatory cells that infiltrate the fibrocalcific plaque.[4–6] The basic mechanism initiating the process of calcification is unknown, but it seems to require apoptosis of intralesional cells, likely smooth muscle cells; the apoptotic bodies would then work as nucleating foci of calcification.

## CALCIUM SCORING AND CARDIOVASCULAR RISK

The tenet of atherosclerosis imaging is that identification of subclinical disease allows early aggressive modification of risk in those at highest risk for future events, with potentially optimal gain. Coronary artery calcium (CAC) is a sensitive indicator of atherosclerosis, and it has been extensively studied for risk stratification of asymptomatic individuals—first, with electron beam CT and, more recently, with multidetector CT scanners (**Figs. 1** and **2**).

Several publications have demonstrated the independent and incremental prognostic value of CAC over traditional risk factors for the prediction of all-cause mortality and cardiovascular events. Shaw and colleagues[7] reported that the adjusted relative risk for all-cause death was 1.64, 1.74, 2.54, and 4.03 for CAC scores of 11 to 100, 101 to 400, 401 to 1000, and greater than 1000, respectively, compared with a CAC score of 1 to 10 in a cohort of 10,377 asymptomatic patients followed for a mean of 5 years. For the prediction of death, the area under the receiver operating characteristic curve (AUC) was greater for CAC than for traditional risk factors (0.72–0.78; $P<.001$).

Greenland and colleagues[8] followed 1312 subjects for a median of 7 years after CAC screening. All patients had at least one risk factor for atherosclerosis, and the primary end point was nonfatal myocardial infarction or CVD.

Division of Cardiology, Department of Medicine, Emory University, 1365 Clifton Road, NE, AT-504, Atlanta, GA 30322, USA
*E-mail address:* praggi@emory.edu

Cardiol Clin 27 (2009) 605–610
doi:10.1016/j.ccl.2009.06.003
0733-8651/09/$ – see front matter 

| Artery | Lesion | Score | Volume | Mean |
|---|---|---|---|---|
| LAD | 11 | 2.89 | 5.92 | 184.89 |
| LAD | 10 | 43.61 | 38.34 | 232.86 |
| LAD | 7 | 2.73 | 5.05 | 159.82 |
| LAD | 6 | 83.04 | 60.76 | 288.59 |
| LAD | 5 | 6.49 | 5.41 | 201.19 |
| LAD | 4 | 6.09 | 7.96 | 193.95 |
| LAD | 2 | 26.45 | 30.56 | 262.74 |
| LAD | 1 | 44.25 | 44.00 | 304.15 |
| LCX | 13 | 21.08 | 21.44 | 258.29 |
| LCX | 12 | 17.63 | 9.21 | 248.93 |
| LCX | 9 | 1.76 | 4.07 | 160.18 |
| LCX | 8 | 21.80 | 22.49 | 223.44 |
| LCX | 3 | 8.66 | 3.55 | 208.81 |
| RCA | 20 | 30.06 | 32.55 | 308.11 |
| RCA | 19 | 26.93 | 15.25 | 292.37 |
| RCA | 18 | 7.86 | 9.17 | 181.24 |
| RCA | 17 | 2.73 | 4.55 | 168.29 |
| RCA | 16 | 3.21 | 6.67 | 182.15 |
| RCA | 15 | 8.58 | 7.49 | 208.68 |
| RCA | 14 | 31.74 | 30.46 | 227.14 |
| Coronaries total | 20 | 397.58 | 364.89 | 252.91 |
| LAD Total | 8 | 215.54 | 198.00 | 264.01 |
| LCX Total | 5 | 70.94 | 60.75 | 231.39 |
| RCA Total | 7 | 111.10 | 106.14 | 248.09 |
| Total: | 20 | **397.58** | 364.89 | 252.91 |

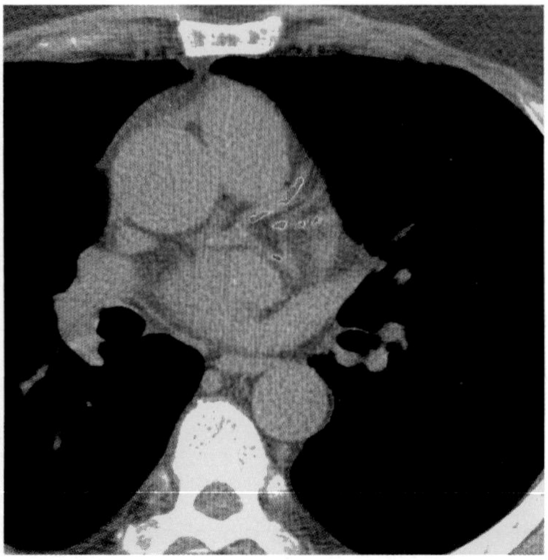

**Fig. 1.** Axial CT images of the chest; CAC in an asymptomatic patient with hypertension and a family history of premature coronary artery disease. The software uses color coding to differentiate plaques seen along the left anterior descending coronary artery (*red*) and circumflex (*blue*) according to the calcium concentration in the plaque (Agatston score = 397.58).

A CAC score greater than 300 was associated with a hazard ratio of 3.9 for the occurrence of a primary event during follow-up. The addition of CAC to traditional risk factors provided incremental prognostic value for the prediction of a cardiac event, although this was true only in patients with a baseline Framingham risk score (FRS) greater than 10% at 10 years.

In the St. Francis Heart Study,[9] 4613 asymptomatic subjects aged 50 to 70 years were followed for 4.3 years after CAC screening. The baseline CAC score was higher in the 119 patients who had cardiovascular events than in those without events (median score [interquartile range]: 384 [127, 800] versus 10 [0, 86]; $P<.0001$). For subjects with a CAC score of 100 or greater versus less than 100, the relative risk (95% confidence interval [CI]) of nonfatal myocardial infarction and death was 9.2 (4.9–17.3). The CAC score predicted cardiovascular events independent of standard risk factors and CRP ($P = .004$) and was superior to the FRS (AUC: 0.79 $\pm$ 0.03 versus 0.69 $\pm$ 0.03; $P = .0006$). Similarly, LaMonte and colleagues,[10] Taylor and colleagues,[11] and Kondos and colleagues[12] added further evidence that CAC works well in intermediate-risk patients to improve risk prediction.

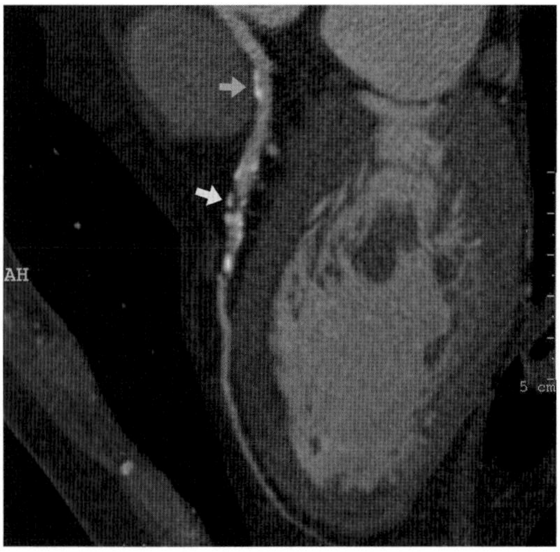


**Fig. 2.** CT coronary angiography shows mixed (*bottom yellow arrow*) and calcified plaques in the left anterior descending artery (*top red arrow*).

## *Calcium Score in Women*

The utility of CAC screening has also been investigated in special subsets of the populations, such as women, diabetic patients, and the elderly. Two original investigations and one meta-analysis supported the utility of CAC for risk stratification in women. The author's group[13] compared the occurrence of all-cause death in approximately 4000 women and 6000 men referred for CAC screening by primary care physicians. CAC scores were lower in women than in men ($P<.0001$), but death rates were higher among older, diabetic, hypertensive, and smoking patients of both genders. In risk-adjusted models, women had a greater probability of death than men for any CAC score. Importantly, CAC added incremental prognostic value to the FRS ($P<.0001$) in both genders.

Lakoski and colleagues[14] conducted gender analyses of the Multi Ethnic Study of Atherosclerosis (MESA) data and noted that a CAC score greater than 0 was a strong predictor of coronary heart and CVD events in 2684 women considered to be at low risk by Framingham categories compared with patients without CAC (hazard ratios of 6.5 and 5.2, respectively). Finally, in a meta-analysis of three prospective and two observational registries, Bellasi and colleagues[15] concluded that CAC screening is equally accurate in stratifying risk for all-cause death and CVD events in women and men.

### *Calcium Score in Diabetic Patients*

Several clinical studies have shown that glucose intolerance and insulin resistance are associated with increased prevalence of CAC[16,17]; similarly, frank diabetes mellitus is associated with a greater extent of CAC compared with that in the nondiabetic population.[18] Wong and colleagues[19] and Anand and colleagues[20] demonstrated an increasing incidence of inducible ischemia on stress myocardial perfusion imaging in diabetic patients with greater amounts of CAC. Type-2 diabetic patients with a CAC score of 10 or less, 11 to 100, 101 to 400, 401 to 1000, and greater than 1000 had an incidence of myocardial ischemia of 0%, 18%, 23%, 48%, and 71%, respectively, and morbidity and mortality increased proportionally with the CAC score and ischemic burden.[20] In an observational registry, Raggi and colleagues[21] showed a higher all-cause mortality rate for any extent of CAC in diabetic subjects than in nondiabetic subjects ($P$>.001). Of interest, the 5-year mortality rate of diabetic patients with little or no CAC (approximately 30% of a cohort of 903 diabetic patients) was as low as that of nondiabetic subjects without CAC (approximately 1% at the end of follow-up).

### *Calcium Score in the Elderly*

CAC maintains its utility as a tool for risk stratification in the elderly. In the prospective Rotterdam study, 2013 participants (mean age: 71 $\pm$ 5.7 years) received CAC screening and measurement of traditional cardiovascular risk factors.[22] Men and women in the highest CAC score category showed an adjusted odds ratio for myocardial infarction of 7.7 (95% CI: 4.1–14.5) and 6.7 (95% CI: 2.4–19.1), respectively, compared with the lowest score category (0–100). The predictive power of CAC was independent of the FRS category (low, intermediate, or high). Raggi and colleagues[23] followed 35,388 patients, with 3570 subjects being 70 years of age or older at screening, for an average period of 5.8 $\pm$ 3 years. The author's group reported an expected increase in all-cause mortality with increasing age (relative hazard per age decile increase = 1.09, 95% CI: 1.08–1.10; $P$<.0001), with higher death rates among men than women (hazard ratio = 1.53, 95% CI: 1.32–1.77; $P$<.0001). Nonetheless, increasing CAC scores were associated with decreasing survival rates across all age deciles ($P$<.0001), suggesting that CAC is predictive even in older age. Finally, using CAC score categories, more than 40% of elderly patients were reclassified to lower or higher risk categories compared with their original FRS group. This was likely the result of a reduction in risk attributed to age, the variable carrying the most weight in the Framingham equations, in the absence of subclinical atherosclerosis.

### *Calcium Score and Ethnicity*

Finally, data from the MESA study and other series[24,25] demonstrated that whites have a higher prevalence of CAC and higher CAC scores than other races, and this raised the question of the validity of CAC in nonwhites. Two recent publications addressed the value of CAC as a marker of risk in four different races (white, African American, Chinese, and Hispanic) in the United States. Nasir and colleagues[25] evaluated the use of CAC to predict all-cause mortality (505 deaths during 10 years of follow-up) in 14,812 patients. The prevalence of CAC was highest in whites, although blacks and Hispanics had a greater clustering of risk factors for CAD. Despite a lower prevalence of CAC and lower scores compared with other races, black patients demonstrated the highest mortality rates even after multivariable adjustment for clinical risk factors and baseline CAC scores ($P$<.0001). Compared with whites, the relative risk for death was 2.97 (95% CI: 1.87–4.72) in blacks, 1.58 (95% CI: 0.92–2.71) in Hispanics, and 0.85 (95% CI: 0.47–1.54) in Chinese. Detrano and colleagues[26] showed that CAC is a strong predictor of CVD, nonfatal myocardial infarction, angina, and revascularization (total events = 162) independent of race in 6722 MESA patients (the risk increased 7.7-fold in patients with a CAC score between 101 and 300 compared with 0- and 9.7-fold in patients with a score >300). Furthermore, CAC added incremental prognostic value beyond traditional risk factors for the prediction of events in all races. Hence, CAC seems to be an excellent marker of risk in all races so far investigated, although the prognostic significance of score categories may vary among racial groups.

The evidence surrounding CAC was recently reviewed in two statements of the American Heart

Association[27] and the American College of Cardiology,[28] which recognized the potential utility of CAC screening for refinement of risk assessment in intermediate-risk patients.

## CONTRAST-ENHANCED CT AND CARDIOVASCULAR RISK

Histopathologic and autopsy studies have demonstrated that CAC amounts to approximately 20% of the total plaque volume. Although the presence of CAC is pathognomonic of the presence of atherosclerosis, its absence on chest CT imaging cannot be taken as absolute proof of absence of atherosclerotic disease. In fact, multiple correlative studies using invasive or noninvasive angiographic techniques have shown that approximately 5% to 8% of patients without CAC may have a critical coronary artery lesion (>50% luminal stenosis).[29,30] This, however, seems to be true particularly in symptomatic patients and may not apply to asymptomatic subjects screened for atherosclerosis.

Numerous investigators have attempted to separate lipid-rich plaques from fibrotic plaques on CT angiography (CTA) by assessing the mean attenuation (density) of areas apparently containing noncalcified plaques and performed comparative studies of CTA and intravascular ultrasound (IVUS). CTA seems to underestimate plaque volume compared with IVUS and shows modest (53%) to good sensitivity (83%) for the identification of noncalcified plaques compared with IVUS. The mean CT attenuation of lipid-rich plaques, which appear hypoechogenic on IVUS, is significantly lower than that of hyperechogenic (ie, fibrotic) plaques, with values ranging from 14 to 58 Hounsfield units (HU) for the former to 90 to 120 HU for the latter.[31–33] CTA performed in patients with acute coronary syndromes shows less CAC or only spotty calcifications, larger and more numerous low-attenuation plaques,[34,35] and positive remodeling compared with the findings of CTA in patients with stable angina. Motoyama and colleagues[36] reported that the simultaneous presence of positive remodeling, areas of low attenuation, and spotty calcification on CTA identifies with 95% accuracy the culprit plaque associated with an acute coronary syndrome. Although attractive, the use of mean attenuation to identify the lipid-rich fracture-prone plaque has a fundamental flaw; most investigators reported a substantial overlap between CT attenuation values of lipid-rich and fibrotic plaques, indicating that relying exclusively on measurement of mean plaque attenuation may not be sufficient to define its vulnerability. Furthermore, there are several other factors to be considered that may temper the enthusiasm for performing CTA in asymptomatic subjects. The presence and degree of luminal stenosis on invasive angiography have not been shown to be predictive of severity and time to events.[37] Furthermore, revascularization of critical stenoses has not been shown to improve survival or reduce the occurrence of myocardial infarction.[38] There is currently no proved and reproducible method to quantify noncalcified plaque burden. A recent study suggested that the incremental value of detecting noncalcified plaque over the simpler CAC score is minimal in asymptomatic patients. In that study, the investigators found coronary atherosclerotic plaques in 215 of 1000 Korean subjects but only 40 (4%) had only noncalcified plaques (calcium score = 0).[39]

Finally, the radiation exposure provided by CTA is high (close to that of a stress nuclear test and greater than that of an uncomplicated diagnostic invasive coronary angiogram). It is therefore logical to conclude that CTA should not be considered a screening tool for refinement of risk prediction in asymptomatic subjects at this time. The American College of Cardiology recently endorsed a list of appropriate uses of CTA, and screening for asymptomatic CAD was excluded.[40]

## FUTURE PERSPECTIVES

Large prospective studies are still needed to ascertain the predictive value of such markers as noncalcified plaque on CTA and plaque composition. The optimal combination of serologic and imaging markers is not clear; at the same time, it is not entirely clear which patients are the most appropriate for screening. In this light, if we limit our scope to the intermediate-risk patients, are we going to underestimate risk in a large portion of patients considered to be at low risk by clinical markers? At the same time, if we only focus on the intermediate-risk patients, are we going to neglect the fact that several high-risk patients may actually be at lower risk? Despite all the obstacles, this remains a viable research venue because one may envision a reduction in large-scale randomized morbidity and mortality trials and an increase in the number of trials based on surrogate outcome measures. Nonetheless, future studies obviously need to concentrate on establishing a correlation between imaging of plaque progression and future cardiovascular events.

## REFERENCES

1. Johnson RC, Leopold JA, Loscalzo J. Vascular calcification: pathobiological mechanisms and clinical implications. Circ Res 2006;99(10):1044–59.

2. Doherty TM, Fitzpatrick LA, Inoue D, et al. Molecular, endocrine, and genetic mechanisms of arterial calcification. Endocr Rev 2004;25(4):629–72.
3. Proudfoot D, Skepper JN, Hegyi L, et al. Apoptosis regulates human vascular calcification in vitro: evidence for initiation of vascular calcification by apoptotic bodies. Circ Res 2000;87(11):1055–62.
4. Doherty TM, Asotra K, Fitzpatrick LA, et al. Calcification in atherosclerosis: bone biology and chronic inflammation at the arterial crossroads. Proc Natl Acad Sci U S A 2003;100(20):11201–6.
5. Aikawa E, Nahrendorf M, Figueiredo JL, et al. Osteogenesis associates with inflammation in early-stage atherosclerosis evaluated by molecular imaging in vivo. Circulation 2007;116(24):2841–50.
6. Qin X, Corriere MA, Matrisian LM, et al. Matrix metalloproteinase inhibition attenuates aortic calcification. Arterioscler Thromb Vasc Biol 2006;26(7): 1510–6.
7. Shaw LJ, Raggi P, Schisterman E, et al. Prognostic value of cardiac risk factors and coronary artery calcium screening for all-cause mortality. Radiology 2003;228(3):826–33.
8. Greenland P, LaBree L, Azen SP, et al. Coronary artery calcium score combined with Framingham score for risk prediction in asymptomatic individuals. JAMA 2004;291(2):210–5.
9. Arad Y, Goodman kJ, Roth M, et al. Coronary calcification, coronary disease risk factors, C-reactive protein, and atherosclerotic cardiovascular disease events: the St. Francis Heart Study. J Am Coll Cardiol 2005;46(1):158–65.
10. LaMonte MJ, FitzGerald SJ, Church TS, et al. Coronary artery calcium score and coronary heart disease events in a large cohort of asymptomatic men and women. Am J Epidemiol 2005;162(5):421–9.
11. Taylor AJ, Bindeman J, Feuerstein I, et al. Coronary calcium independently predicts incident premature coronary heart disease over measured cardiovascular risk factors: mean three-year outcomes in the Prospective Army Coronary Calcium (PACC) project. J Am Coll Cardiol 2005;46(5):807–14.
12. Kondos GT, Hoff JA, Sevrukov A, et al. Electron-beam tomography coronary artery calcium and cardiac events: a 37-month follow-up of 5635 initially asymptomatic low- to intermediate-risk adults. Circulation 2003;107(20):2571–6.
13. Raggi P, Shaw LJ, Berman DS, et al. Gender-based differences in the prognostic value of coronary calcification. J Womens Health (Larchmt) 2004;13(3): 273–83.
14. Lakoski SG, Greenland P, Wong ND, et al. Coronary artery calcium scores and risk for cardiovascular events in women classified as "low risk" based on Framingham risk score: the Multi-Ethnic Study of Atherosclerosis (MESA). Arch Intern Med 2007; 167(22):2437–42.
15. Bellasi A, Lacey C, Taylor AJ, et al. Comparison of prognostic usefulness of coronary artery calcium in men versus women (results from a meta- and pooled analysis estimating all-cause mortality and coronary heart disease death or myocardial infarction). Am J Cardiol 2007;100(3):409–14.
16. Dabelea D, Kinney G, Snell-Bergeon JK, et al. Effect of type 1 diabetes on the gender difference in coronary artery calcification: a role for insulin resistance? The Coronary Artery Calcification in Type 1 Diabetes (CACTI) Study. Diabetes 2003; 52(11):2833–9.
17. Meigs JB, Larson MG, D'Agostino RB, et al. Coronary artery calcification in type 2 diabetes and insulin resistance: the Framingham Offspring Study. Diabetes Care 2002;25(8):1313–9.
18. Wong ND, Sciammarella MG, Polk D, et al. The metabolic syndrome, diabetes, and subclinical atherosclerosis assessed by coronary calcium. J Am Coll Cardiol 2003;41(9):1547–53.
19. Wong ND, Rozanski A, Gransar H, et al. Metabolic syndrome and diabetes are associated with an increased likelihood of inducible myocardial ischemia among patients with subclinical atherosclerosis. Diabetes Care 2005;28(6):1445–50.
20. Anand DV, Lim E, Hopkins D, et al. Risk stratification in uncomplicated type 2 diabetes: prospective evaluation of the combined use of coronary artery calcium imaging and selective myocardial perfusion scintigraphy. Eur Heart J 2006;27(6): 713–21.
21. Raggi P, Shaw LJ, Berman DS, et al. Prognostic value of coronary artery calcium screening in subjects with and without diabetes. J Am Coll Cardiol 2004;43(9):1663–9.
22. Vliegenthart R, Oudkerk M, Hofman A, et al. Coronary calcification improves cardiovascular risk prediction in the elderly. Circulation 2005;112(4): 572–7.
23. Raggi P, Gongora MC, Gopal A, et al. Coronary artery calcium to predict all-cause mortality in elderly men and women. J Am Coll Cardiol 2008;52(1):17–23.
24. Bild DE, Detrano R, Peterson D, et al. Ethnic differences in coronary calcification: the Multi-Ethnic Study of Atherosclerosis (MESA). Circulation 2005; 111(10):1313–20.
25. Nasir K, Shaw LJ, Liu ST, et al. Ethnic differences in the prognostic value of coronary artery calcification for all-cause mortality. J Am Coll Cardiol 2007; 50(10):953–60.
26. Detrano R, Guerci AD, Carr JJ, et al. Coronary calcium as a predictor of coronary events in four racial or ethnic groups. N Engl J Med 2008; 358(13):1336–45.
27. Budoff MJ, Achenbach S, Blumenthal RS, et al. Assessment of coronary artery disease by cardiac

computed tomography: a scientific statement from the American Heart Association Committee on Cardiovascular Imaging and Intervention, Council on Cardiovascular Radiology and Intervention, and Committee on Cardiac Imaging, Council on Clinical Cardiology. Circulation 2006;114(16):1761–91.

28. Greenland P, Bonow RO, Brundage BH, et al. ACCF/AHA 2007 clinical expert consensus document on coronary artery calcium scoring by computed tomography in global cardiovascular risk assessment and in evaluation of patients with chest pain: a report of the American College of Cardiology Foundation Clinical Expert Consensus Task Force (ACCF/AHA Writing Committee to Update the 2000 Expert Consensus Document on Electron Beam Computed Tomography) developed in collaboration with the Society of Atherosclerosis Imaging and Prevention and the Society of Cardiovascular Computed Tomography. J Am Coll Cardiol 2007; 49(3):378–402.
29. Becker A, Leber A, White CW, et al. Multislice computed tomography for determination of coronary artery disease in a symptomatic patient population. Int J Cardiovasc Imaging 2007;23(3):361–7.
30. Cheng VY, Lepor NE, Madyoon H, et al. Presence and severity of noncalcified coronary plaque on 64-slice computed tomographic coronary angiography in patients with zero and low coronary artery calcium. Am J Cardiol 2007;99(9):1183–6.
31. Leber AW, Knez A, Becker A, et al. Accuracy of multidetector spiral computed tomography in identifying and differentiating the composition of coronary atherosclerotic plaques: a comparative study with intracoronary ultrasound. J Am Coll Cardiol 2004; 43(7):1241–7.
32. Schroeder S, Kopp AF, Baumbach A, et al. Noninvasive detection and evaluation of atherosclerotic coronary plaques with multislice computed tomography. J Am Coll Cardiol 2001;37(5):1430–5.
33. Pohle K, Achenbach S, Macneill B, et al. Characterization of non-calcified coronary atherosclerotic plaque by multi-detector row CT: comparison to IVUS. Atherosclerosis 2007;190(1):174–80.
34. Leber AW, Knez A, White CW, et al. Composition of coronary atherosclerotic plaques in patients with acute myocardial infarction and stable angina pectoris determined by contrast-enhanced multislice computed tomography. Am J Cardiol 2003;91(6): 714–8.
35. Schuijf JD, Beck T, Burgstahler C, et al. Differences in plaque composition and distribution in stable coronary artery disease versus acute coronary syndromes; non-invasive evaluation with multi-slice computed tomography. Acute Card Care 2007; 9(1):48–53.
36. Motoyama S, Kondo T, Sarai M, et al. Multislice computed tomographic characteristics of coronary lesions in acute coronary syndromes. J Am Coll Cardiol 2007;50(4):319–26.
37. Ambrose JA, Tannenbaum MA, Alexopoulos D, et al. Angiographic progression of coronary artery disease and the development of myocardial infarction. J Am Coll Cardiol 1988;12(1):56–62.
38. Boden WE, O'Rourke RA, Teo KK, et al. Optimal medical therapy with or without PCI for stable coronary disease. N Engl J Med 2007;356(15): 1503–16.
39. Choi EK, Choi SI, Rivera JJ, et al. Coronary computed tomography angiography as a screening tool for the detection of occult coronary artery disease in asymptomatic individuals. J Am Coll Cardiol 2008;52:357–65.
40. Hendel RC, Patel MR, Kramer CM, et al. ACCF/ACR/SCCT/SCMR/ASNC/NASCI/SCAI/SIR 2006 appropriateness criteria for cardiac computed tomography and cardiac magnetic resonance imaging: a report of the American College of Cardiology Foundation Quality Strategic Directions Committee Appropriateness Criteria Working Group, American College of Radiology, Society of Cardiovascular Computed Tomography, Society for Cardiovascular Magnetic Resonance, American Society of Nuclear Cardiology, North American Society for Cardiac Imaging, Society for Cardiovascular Angiography and Interventions, and Society of Interventional Radiology. J Am Coll Cardiol 2006;48(7):1475–97.

# Evaluation of Coronary Atherosclerotic Plaques

Christoph R. Becker, MD*, Tobias Saam, MD

**KEYWORDS**

• CT • MRI • Coronary calcium • Vulnerable plaque
• Coronary CT angiography

Coronary atherosclerosis begins as early as in the first decade of life, with endothelia dysfunction, proliferation of smooth muscle cells, and accumulation of fat (fatty streaks) in the coronary artery wall.[1] At the later stage of the disease, these lesions may accumulate cholesterol within the intimal and media layer of the coronary artery wall, with a fibrous cap separating the lipid pool from the coronary artery lumen.[2] Inflammatory processes with invasion of macrophages and activation of matrix metalloproteinases cause consecutive weakening of the fibrous cap.[3] At the same time, inflammation may lead to weakening of the coronary artery wall with consecutive widening of the outer wall. This phenomenon is called positive remodeling and may be the reason that often such plaques may be missed by conventional invasive coronary angiography.[4]

Vulnerable plaques may rupture when exposed to shear stress, and thrombogenic lipid material may get contact to the blood. In the most unfortunate event, thrombus progression may turn the vulnerable plaque into a culprit lesion that occludes the coronary vessel, leading to myocardial ischemia, ventricular fibrillation, and death.[5] Chronic nonfatal plaque rupture and healing may result in fibro-calcified lesions that lead to negative remodeling with shrinking of the vessel lumen, leading to myocardial ischemia. Therefore acute coronary events and unheralded myocardial infarction more often are associated with vulnerable plaques, whereas stable angina more often is associated with stable plaques.

## EPIDEMIOLOGY OF CORONARY ATHEROSCLEROSIS

In many patients, unheralded myocardial infarction associated with a mortality of approximately 20% is the first manifestation of coronary artery disease (CAD). The risk of an event strongly depends on risk factors, such as hypertension, hypercholesteremia, smoking, family history, age, and gender. Based of these risk factors, the Framingham[6] and Prospective Cardiovascular Münster Study (PROCAM)[7] algorithms provide an estimation of the midterm (10-year) risk for an individual to experience a cardiac event. According to international guidelines, subjects who have a midterm risk of less than 10% are considered to be at low risk and usually do not require any specific therapy. Patients who have a midterm risk of more than 20% are considered to be at high risk and therefore may be considered as subjects with a CAD equivalent. Similar to patients who have established CAD, these asymptomatic subjects may require intensive therapy such as lifestyle changes and lifetime medical treatment.

Approximately 40% of the population is considered to have a moderate midterm risk of 10% to 20%. Any of the stratification schemes suffers from a lack of accuracy to correctly determine the risk, and uncertainty exists as to how to treat subjects who have been identified to be at intermediate risk. Other tools providing information about the necessity to either reassure or to treat these subjects are warranted. Currently, the assessment of the atherosclerotic plaque burden

Department of Clinical Radiology, Ludwig-Maximilians-University Munich, Grosshadern Clinics, Marchioninistraße 15, 81377 Munich, Germany
* Corrresponding author.
*E-mail address:* christoph.becker@med.uni-muenchen.de (C.R. Becker).

Cardiol Clin 27 (2009) 611–617
doi:10.1016/j.ccl.2009.06.013
0733-8651/09/$ – see front matter 

by CT may be able provide valid information for this cohort.[8]

## NONINVASIVE EVALUATION OF ATHEROSCLEROTIC PLAQUE COMPONENTS

### *Calcium Scoring*

Coronary calcium is a surrogate marker for coronary atherosclerosis. Levels of coronary calcium have been measured by electron beam computed tomography (EBCT) for more than a decade. Several prospective cohort studies are underway to assess whether coronary calcium evaluation is superior to assessing conventional risk factors when estimating the risk of future cardiovascular events. Initial results published from the South Bay Heart Watch study (2000 subjects) show that coronary calcium is of minor predictive value in patients who have diabetes, and that differences exist in terms of prevalence and progression of coronary calcium in different ethnic groups.[9] The Heinz-Nixdorf risk factors, evaluation of coronary calcium, and lifestyle (RECALL) study (4200 subjects) provides unbiased information on the extent of coronary calcium in the general German population from a suburban community.[10]

The authors of the Prospective Army Coronary Calcium study (2000, 40- to 50-year-olds) found the CT-based assessment of coronary calcium to be superior to the conventional Framingham risk score when determining the risk of future cardiac events. Similar predictive value has been found for individuals who have coronary calcium and a positive family history of coronary heart disease. The high cost of EBCT may have contributed to the calculated amount of $37,633 per quality-adjusted life year saved (QALY). In other words, screening for CAD under these circumstances yet does not seem to be cost-effective.[11]

The Multi Ethnic Study of Atherosclerosis (MESA) (6800 subjects) has reported that all modern multidetector row CT systems are at least as reliable as EBCT for performing and reproducing coronary calcium measurements.[12] In this study, again the coronary calcium score was superior to conventional risk factors for predicting coronary heart disease. This was true even for all four major racial and ethnic groups in the United States.[13] Further studies are needed to determine whether coronary calcium screening performed by MSCT is a cost-effective option for risk stratification and preventing of unheralded myocardial infarction in certain selected patient populations.

### *Contrast-Enhanced CT Angiography*

Coronary CT angiography (CTA) has a high negative predictive value for stenotic CAD as compared with cardiac catheterization (discussed further in the article by Thompson in this issue). In patients who have unspecific complaints or ambiguous stress tests, CTA may serve as a reliable noninvasive alternative to rule out CAD. More than only displaying the contrast-filled lumen like in cardiac catheterization, CTA as a cross-sectional modality also has the ability to display the coronary artery wall. Coronary atherosclerotic changes may appear as calcified, noncalcified, or mixed plaques. Noncalcified lesions are found predominantly in patients who have acute myocardial infarction, whereas calcified lesions are found more often in patients who have chronic stable angina.[14] The CT density of noncalcified plaques is significantly lower in the culprit coronary segment of patients studied at the time of acute coronary syndromes as compared with those who have chronic stable disease.[15] In patients who have an acute coronary syndrome, a noncalcified lesion in the coronary artery may correspond to an intracoronary thrombus.[16]

The current gold standard to detect coronary atherosclerosis in vivo is intravascular ultrasound (IVUS). Studies comparing IVUS with multidetector row CT (MDCT) have shown a good correlation between the echogenicity by IVUS and the CT density of coronary atherosclerotic lesions.[17] The sensitivity and specificity for CT to detect calcified and noncalcified coronary atherosclerosis are 78% and 94%, respectively. The sensitivity to detect noncalcified plaques in a lesion-by-lesion comparison between CTA and IVUS is only 52%,[18] however, probably because of the lower spatial resolution if CTA. **Figs. 1** and **2** are CTA images of typical calcified and noncalcified coronary plaques.

CT density measurement in carotid arteries[19] and heart specimen[20] has shown that mean CT attenuation values around 50 hounsfield units (HU) and 90 HU within plaques are specific for lipid and fibrous tissues, respectively. In work done by Langheinrich and colleagues with micro-CT and ultrahigh spatial resolution, the ability of CT to distinguish between different plaque components such as lipid, fibrin, and calcium within a plaque has been demonstrated. Interestingly, the proliferation of smooth muscle cells also increases the CT density of the plaque.[21]

Recently, the authors observed a plaque in a patient with unstable angina who developed a myocardial infarction in due course with a culprit lesion at the location of the former plaque. The vulnerable plaque that had been detected before its rupture had a dark center surrounded by a bright rim, most likely corresponding to a lipid pool and a fibrous cap, respectively.

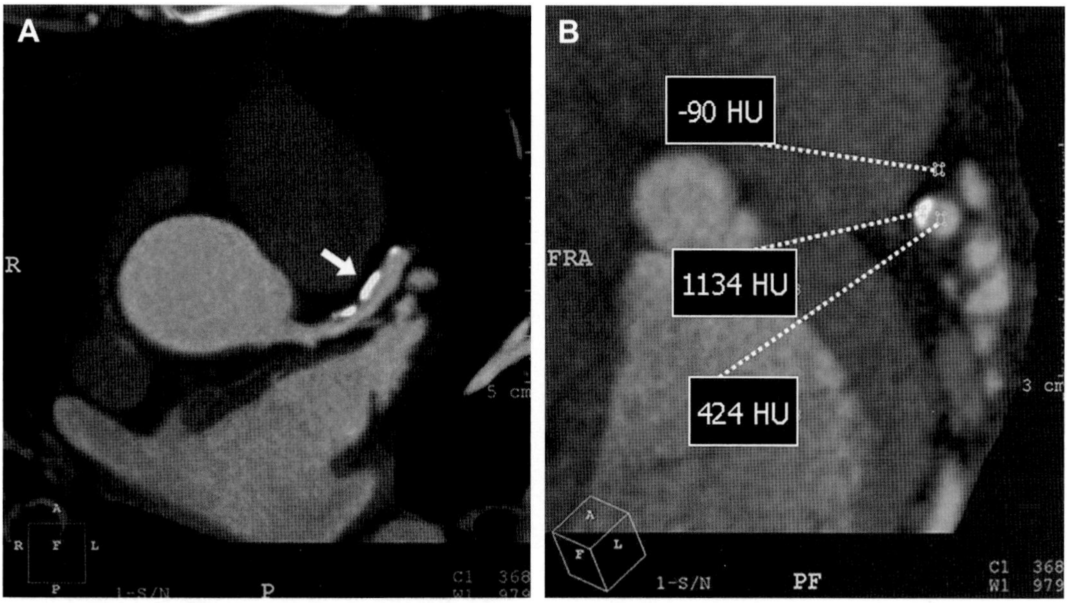


**Fig. 1.** Axial (*A*) and oblique cross-sectional (*B*) views of a calcified atherosclerotic coronary plaque associated with mild luminal obstruction in the mid- left anterior coronary artery. The mean attenuation of the plaque is 1134 HU, compared with the contrast-enhanced lumen (424 HU) and epicardial fat (-90 HU).

## *MRI*

MRI has unique potential to identify the key features of the vulnerable plaque. The excellent soft tissue contrast provided by MRI allows evaluation of compositional and morphologic features of carotid atherosclerotic plaques.[22] In particular, it has been shown that in vivo carotid MRI is able to identify and to quantify the lipid-rich/necrotic core, calcification, hemorrhage, thrombus, and the fibrous cap with good correlation to histopathology.[22–24] Furthermore MRI is noninvasive,

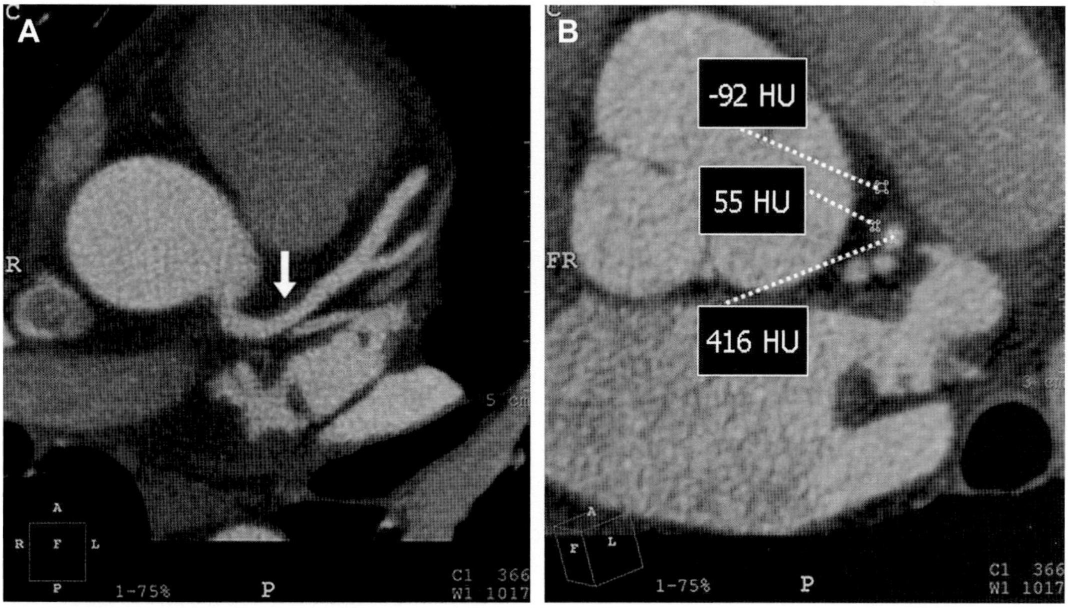


**Fig. 2.** Axial (*A*) and oblique cross-sectional views (*B*) of a noncalcified atherosclerotic coronary plaque associated with mild luminal obstruction in the proximal left anterior coronary artery. The mean attenuation of the plaque is 55 HU, compared with the contrast-enhanced lumen (416 HU) and epicardial fat (-92 HU).

does not involve ionizing radiation, enables the visualization of the vessel lumen and wall,[25,26] and can be repeated serially to track progression or regression. Most of the MRI studies, however, have been performed in carotid arteries. The carotid arteries are superficial and stationary vessels with a relatively large diameter and therefore ideally suited for MRI with dedicated surface coils. In contrast, noninvasive MRI of the coronary arteries is a formidable task. The small diameter of the coronary arteries (approximately 2 to 4 mm), their tortuous course, their close anatomic relationship to the coronary veins and cardiac chambers, and finally, their continuous, rapid motion caused by cardiac contraction and respiratory excursions create obstacles that are difficult to overcome.

Kim and colleagues[27] used a free-breathing, navigator-gated, three-dimensional magnetic resonance (MR) technique to visualize the coronary arteries and to detect coronary stenoses in a series of 109 patients. In segments that could be evaluated, 78 of 94 stenoses greater than 50% were detected by MR angiography (MRA) using invasive coronary angiography as the gold standard. In a separate analysis, the authors calculated a sensitivity of 100% for identifying either left main CAD or three-vessel disease, conditions in which revascularization is of particular therapeutic value. Current spatial (approximately 1 × 1 × 2 mm) and temporal resolution (approximately 60 to 125 milliseconds), however, permits imaging only in the proximal two thirds of the coronary arteries and exclusive of the major side branches.[28] Although coronary MR angiography (MRA) is promising, further development is needed before routine clinical use.[28] Recently, alternative acquisition techniques have been proposed,[29] establishing different contrast behavior, such as with steady-state free precession (SSFP) techniques,[30] and using different k-space acquisition schemes, such as spiral[31] or radial (also known as projection–reconstruction)[32] readout patterns. Furthermore, a whole-heart SSFP coronary MRA technique has been proposed[29] that improves visible vessel length and facilitates high-quality coronary MRA of the complete coronary tree in a single measurement. These newer sequences were reported to provide several advantages over the free-breathing, T2-prepared segmented gradient echo (SGE) sequences,[33,34] including increased signal-to-noise ratio, contrast-to-noise ratio, vessel sharpness, and vessel length, and reduced acquisition time.

Besides providing information of the arterial lumen, MRI is able to visualize the full vessel wall. In a study including six healthy subjects and six subjects who had nonsignificant CAD (10% to 50% radiograph angiographic diameter reduction), Kim and colleagues[35] introduced a noninvasive MRI method to detect expansive remodeling in coronary arteries. Free-breathing three-dimensional black blood coronary cardiac MR (CMR) with isotropic resolution identified an increased coronary vessel wall thickness with preservation of lumen size in patients who had nonsignificant CAD, consistent with an expansive arterial remodeling. A recent study in 15 volunteers demonstrated the feasibility of coronary wall imaging using free breathing and breath hold two-dimensional black blood turbo spin echo (TSE) at 3T.[36] Although measurements of coronary wall thickness, wall area, lumen diameter, and lumen area were consistent with previous MR measurements at 1.5T, the authors concluded that further improvement in resolution and image quality is required to detect and characterize coronary plaques.[36] In one of the largest clinical coronary MRI studies to date,[37] 136 subjects who had long-standing type 1 diabetes without symptoms or history of cardiovascular disease, including 63 patients (46%) who had nephropathy and 73 patients who normo-albuminuria, underwent cardiovascular MRI. The study showed that in asymptomatic type 1 diabetes, cardiovascular magnetic resonance imaging reveals greater coronary plaque burden - expressed as right coronary artery mean wall thickness - in subjects with nephropathy compared with those with normo-albuminuria.

More recent studies have examined the usefulness of contrast media application for further characterization of the coronary vessel wall. In a study[38] with 14 patients who had cardiovascular risk factors and 6 healthy subjects without risk factors, delayed-enhancement cardiovascular MR (DE-CMR) coronary artery wall imaging was performed and compared with MDCT and quantitative coronary angiography (QCA). The authors showed a higher prevalence of delayed enhancement in more diseased arterial segments as assessed by multi-detector-row CT (MDCT) or QCA. Maintz and colleagues[39] evaluated the utility of a T1 weighted black blood inversion recovery coronary MRI sequence before and after administration of gadolinium (Gd)-diethylenetriamene pentaacetate (DTPA) for selective visualization and noninvasive differentiation of atherosclerotic coronary plaque in nine patients who had CAD as confirmed by invasive angiography and MDCT. On contrast-enhanced MRI, 13 of 29 (45%) plaques, 11 of which were mixed, 1 noncalcified, and 1 calcified, showed contrast uptake. All others remained dark. The authors concluded that the observed contrast uptake may be associated with endothelial dysfunction, neovascularization, inflammation, or fibrosis. Although these initial reports with gadolinium contrast agents are promising, further studies are needed to evaluate the usefulness of contrast- enhanced MRI for coronary wall imaging.

Recent research has focused on the development of new targeted contrast agents, which are able to detect local small thrombi.[40] Fibrin can be identified by lipid-encapsulated perfluorocarbon paramagnetic nanoparticles in vitro[41] and in vivo.[42] Botnar and colleagues[43] used a fibrin-binding gadolinium-labeled peptide in an experimental rabbit animal model of plaque rupture and thrombosis to detect acute and subacute thrombosis. Similar agents have been used successfully in swine to detect coronary thrombus and in-stent thrombosis[44] and to detect pulmonary emboli.[45] An initial phase 2 trial in people of molecular MRI[46] enrolled 11 patients who had thrombus in the left ventricle (n=2), left or right atrium (n=4), thoracic aorta (n=4) or carotid artery (n=1) to test the usefulness of a new fibrin-specific contrast agent (EP-2104R, EPIX Pharmaceuticals, Lexington, MA, USA) for improved visualization of thrombi. On enhanced images, thrombi demonstrated high signal amplification, typically at the clot surface, with a significantly increased contrast compared with the surrounding blood pool and soft tissue. The authors concluded that EP-2104R allows for molecular MRI of thrombi potentially responsible for stroke.

## FUTURE TECHNICAL AND CLINICAL POTENTIALS

Although findings of recent studies appear promising, several challenges remain in MRI. Most of the in vivo MR studies in people are based on analysis of data from relatively large human vessels, such as the carotid arteries. To achieve similar results in the much smaller coronary arteries, significant advances in temporal and spatial resolution are necessary. This may be accomplished with improvements in pulse sequence design and MR hardware (eg, higher-field MRI, coil design).

If the ability of coronary CTA holds true to detect vulnerable plaques in patients who have acute coronary syndrome directly, new strategies need to be considered for appropriate treatment of these patients. The noninvasive vulnerable plaque detection may justify intensive medical treatment or may lead to invasive approaches such as plaque sealing.

In patients who have atypical chest pain, CTA soon may serve as a tool for complete diagnostic work-up. A CTA investigation may allow ruling in or out pulmonary emboli, aortic dissection, or coronary thrombus with one single scan. Currently however, it appears unlikely that coronary CTA may be used as a screening tool for vulnerable plaques in asymptomatic subjects because of the necessity to administer contrast media and the comparably high radiation exposure for this application.

Some technical improvements of MDCT are foreseeable within the next few years, such as shorter exposure times and higher spatial resolution. Exposure times will become short enough to scan the coronary arteries at any heart rate without the necessity to administer beta-blockers, and the higher spatial resolution will reduce the artifact caused by metal or calcium. Once theses requirements are fulfilled, coronary CTA may replace invasive angiography for triaging patients for conservative, interventional, or surgical therapy, and may reduce the use of an invasive diagnostic procedure on preselected patients in whom coronary interventions are required.

Plaque imaging, and in particular the detection of vulnerable plaques in the coronary arteries, will remain a challenge for CT, because the size of these lesions is in the range of the physical limit for CT. The quantification of coronary atherosclerosis therefore remains a difficult task, and reproducibility will suffer from the low spatial resolution. Furthermore, apart from the morphology, CTA alone may not be able to provide further information about inflammation and shear stress for any plaque detected. Therefore, the only currently foreseeable clinical application for plaque imaging by CTA may be the detection of culprit lesions in the coronary arteries of patients suffering from unstable angina. CTA for acute chest pain already has become clinical routine, because this protocol provides information about potential differential diagnoses apart from CAD.[47] The reliability of CT to detect culprit plaques in this scenario remains the topic of future research, and accordingly, strategies need to be developed to treat these patients once such plaques are detected.

## REFERENCES

1. Stary HC, Chandler AB, Glagov S, et al. A definition of initial, fatty streak, and intermediate lesions of atherosclerosis. A report from the Committee on Vascular Lesions of the Council on Arteriosclerosis, American Heart Association. Circulation 1994;89:2462–78.
2. Stary HC, Chandler AB, Dinsmore RE, et al. A definition of advanced types of atherosclerotic lesions and a histological classification of atherosclerosis. A report from the Committee on Vascular Lesions of

the Council on Arteriosclerosis, American Heart Association. Circulation 1995;92:1355–74.
3. Pasterkamp G, Falk E, Woutman H, et al. Techniques characterizing the coronary atherosclerotic plaque: influence on clinical decision making? J Am Coll Cardiol 2000;36:13–21.
4. Glagov S, Weisenberg E, Zarins C, et al. Compensatory enlargement of human atherosclerotic coronary arteries. N Engl J Med 1987;316:1371–5.
5. Virmani R, Kolodgie FD, Burke AP, et al. Lessons from sudden coronary death. A comprehensive morphological classification scheme for atherosclerotic lesions. Arterioscler Thromb Vasc Biol 2000; 20:1262–75.
6. Wilson PW, D'Agostino RB, Levy D, et al. Prediction of coronary heart disease using risk factor categories. Circulation 1998;97:1837–47.
7. Assmann G, Cullen P, Schulte H. Simple scoring scheme for calculating the risk of acute coronary events based on the 10-year follow-up of the Prospective Cardiovascular Munster (PROCAM) study. Circulation 2002;105:310–5.
8. Greenland P, Abrams J, Aurigemma GP, et al. Prevention Conference V: beyond secondary prevention. Identifying the high-risk patient for primary prevention: noninvasive tests of atherosclerotic burden. Writing Group III. Circulation 2000; 101:E16–22.
9. Greenland P, LaBree L, Azen SP, et al. Coronary artery calcium score combined with Framingham score for risk prediction in asymptomatic individuals. JAMA 2004;291:210–5.
10. Schmermund A, Mohlenkamp S, Berenbein S, et al. Population-based assessment of subclinical coronary atherosclerosis using electron-beam computed tomography. Atherosclerosis 2006;185: 177–82.
11. Taylor AJ, Bindeman J, Feuerstein I, et al. Coronary calcium independently predicts incident premature coronary heart disease over measured cardiovascular risk factors: mean three-year outcomes in the Prospective Army Coronary Calcium (PACC) project. J Am Coll Cardiol 2005;46:807–14.
12. Detrano RC, Anderson M, Nelson J, et al. Coronary calcium measurements: effect of CT scanner type and calcium measure on rescan reproducibility—MESA study. Radiology 2005;236:477–84.
13. Detrano R, Guerci AD, Carr JJ, et al. Coronary calcium as a predictor of coronary events in four racial or ethnic groups. N Engl J Med 2008;358: 1336–45.
14. Leber AW, Knez A, White CW, et al. Composition of coronary atherosclerotic plaques in patients with acute myocardial infarction and stable angina pectoris determined by contrast-enhanced multislice computed tomography. Am J Cardiol 2003;91: 714–8.
15. Inoue F, Sato Y, Matsumoto N, et al. Evaluation of plaque texture by means of multislice computed tomography in patients with acute coronary syndrome and stable angina. Circ J 2004;68:840–4.
16. Becker CR, Knez A, Ohnesorge B, et al. Imaging of noncalcified coronary plaques using helical CT with retrospective ECG gating. AJR Am J Roentgenol 2000;175:423–4.
17. Schroeder S, Kopp AF, Baumbach A, et al. Noninvasive detection of coronary lesions by multislice computed tomography: results of the new age pilot trial. Catheter Cardiovasc Interv 2001;53: 352–8.
18. Achenbach S, Moselewski F, Ropers D, et al. Detection of calcified and noncalcified coronary atherosclerotic plaque by contrast-enhanced, submillimeter multidetector spiral computed tomography: a segment-based comparison with intravascular ultrasound. Circulation 2004;109:14–7.
19. Estes J, Quist W, Lo Gerfo F, et al. Noninvasive characterization of plaque morphology using helical computed tomography. J Cardiovasc Surg 1998; 39:527–34.
20. Becker CR, Nikolaou K, Muders M, et al. Ex vivo coronary atherosclerotic plaque characterization with multidetector row CT. Eur Radiol 2003;13: 2094–8.
21. Langheinrich AC, Bohle RM, Greschus S, et al. Atherosclerotic lesions at micro-CT: feasibility for analysis of coronary artery wall in autopsy specimens. Radiology 2004;231:675–81.
22. Saam T, Hatsukami TS, Takaya N, et al. The vulnerable, or high-risk, atherosclerotic plaque: noninvasive MR imaging for characterization and assessment. Radiology 2007;244:64–77.
23. Cai J, Hatsukami TS, Ferguson MS, et al. In vivo quantitative measurement of intact fibrous cap and lipid-rich necrotic core size in atherosclerotic carotid plaque: comparison of high-resolution, contrast-enhanced magnetic resonance imaging and histology. Circulation 2005;112:3437–44.
24. Saam T, Ferguson MS, Yarnykh VL, et al. Quantitative evaluation of carotid plaque composition by in vivo MRI. Arterioscler Thromb Vasc Biol 2005;25: 234–9.
25. Choudhury RP, Fuster V, Badimon JJ, et al. MRI and characterization of atherosclerotic plaque: emerging applications and molecular imaging. Arterioscler Thromb Vasc Biol 2002;22:1065–74.
26. Yuan C, Mitsumori LM, Beach KW, et al. Carotid atherosclerotic plaque: noninvasive MR characterization and identification of vulnerable lesions. Radiology 2001;221:285–99.
27. Kim WY, Danias PG, Stuber M, et al. Coronary magnetic resonance angiography for the detection of coronary stenoses. N Engl J Med 2001;345: 1863–9.

28. Ropers D, Regenfus M, Wasmeier G, et al. Noninterventional cardiac diagnostics: computed tomography, magnetic resonance and real-time three-dimensional echocardiography. Techniques and clinical applications. Minerva Cardioangiol 2004;52:407–17.
29. Weber OM, Pujadas S, Martin AJ, et al. Free-breathing, three-dimensional coronary artery magnetic resonance angiography: comparison of sequences. J Magn Reson Imaging 2004;20: 395–402.
30. Deshpande VS, Shea SM, Laub G, et al. 3D magnetization-prepared true-FISP: a new technique for imaging coronary arteries. Magn Reson Med 2001; 46:494–502.
31. Bornert P, Stuber M, Botnar RM, et al. Direct comparison of 3D spiral vs. Cartesian gradient echo coronary magnetic resonance angiography. Magn Reson Med 2001;46:789–94.
32. Katoh M, Stuber M, Buecker A, et al. Spin labeling coronary MR angiography with steady-state free precession and radial k-space sampling: initial results in healthy volunteers. Radiology 2005;236:1047–52.
33. Botnar RM, Stuber M, Danias PG, et al. Improved coronary artery definition with T2 weighted, free-breathing, three-dimensional coronary MRA. Circulation 1999;99:3139–48.
34. Stuber M, Botnar RM, Danias PG, et al. Double-oblique free-breathing high resolution three-dimensional coronary magnetic resonance angiography. J Am Coll Cardiol 1999;34:524–31.
35. Kim WY, Stuber M, Bornert P, et al. Three-dimensional black blood cardiac magnetic resonance coronary vessel wall imaging detects positive arterial remodeling in patients with nonsignificant coronary artery disease. Circulation 2002;106:296–9.
36. Koktzoglou I, Simonetti O, Li D. Coronary artery wall imaging: initial experience at 3 Tesla. J Magn Reson Imaging 2005;21:128–32.
37. Kim WY, Astrup AS, Stuber M, et al. Subclinical coronary and aortic atherosclerosis detected by magnetic resonance imaging in type 1 diabetes with and without diabetic nephropathy. Circulation 2007;115:228–35.
38. Yeon SB, Sabir A, Clouse M, et al. Delayed-enhancement cardiovascular magnetic resonance coronary artery wall imaging: comparison with multislice computed tomography and quantitative coronary angiography. J Am Coll Cardiol 2007;50:441–7.
39. Maintz D, Ozgun M, Hoffmeier A, et al. Selective coronary artery plaque visualization and differentiation by contrast-enhanced inversion prepared MRI. Eur Heart J 2006;27:1732–6.
40. Wentzel JJ, Aguiar SH, Fayad ZA. Vascular MRI in the diagnosis and therapy of the high-risk atherosclerotic plaque. J Interv Cardiol 2003;16:129–42.
41. Yu X, Song SK, Chen J, et al. High-resolution MRI characterization of human thrombus using a novel fibrin-targeted paramagnetic nanoparticle contrast agent. Magn Reson Med 2000;44:867–72.
42. Flacke S, Fischer S, Scott MJ, et al. Novel MRI contrast agent for molecular imaging of fibrin: implications for detecting vulnerable plaques. Circulation 2001;104:1280–5.
43. Botnar RM, Perez AS, Witte S, et al. In vivo molecular imaging of acute and subacute thrombosis using a fibrin-binding magnetic resonance imaging contrast agent. Circulation 2004;109:2023–9.
44. Botnar RM, Buecker A, Wiethoff AJ, et al. In vivo magnetic resonance imaging of coronary thrombosis using a fibrin-binding molecular magnetic resonance contrast agent. Circulation 2004;110:1463–6.
45. Spuentrup E, Fausten B, Kinzel S, et al. Molecular magnetic resonance imaging of atrial clots in a swine model. Circulation 2005;112:396–9.
46. Spuentrup E, Botnar RM, Wiethoff AJ, et al. MR imaging of thrombi using EP-2104R, a fibrin-specific contrast agent: initial results in patients. Eur Radiol 2008;18:1995–2005.
47. White CS, Kuo D, Kelemen M, et al. Chest pain evaluation in the emergency department: can MDCT provide a comprehensive evaluation? AJR Am J Roentgenol 2005;185:533–40.

# CT Applications in Electrophysiology

Subodh B. Joshi, MBBS[a], Andrew R. Blum, MD[a], Moussa Mansour, MD[b], Suhny Abbara, MD[a,*]

**KEYWORDS**

- CT • Electrophysiology • Radiofrequency ablation
- Cardiac resynchronization therapy • Cardiac imaging

Over recent years, there have been extraordinary advances in the management of cardiac arrhythmias. Increasingly complex procedures are being performed, and the breadth of conditions for which invasive arrhythmia therapy is indicated continues to grow. In addition to atrial and ventricular ablation procedures for treating arrhythmias, implantable defibrillators and biventricular pacemakers for cardiac resynchronization therapy have made electrophysiology (EP) an important part of heart failure management.[1–4]

As electrophysiology has advanced, the need for high-quality cardiac imaging also has become greater. Detailed anatomical information is required for procedure planning, to improve procedural efficiency, and to monitor for complications. Although echocardiography remains crucial, CT rapidly is becoming an integral part of patient management.[5] In a single 1- to 15-second acquisition, cardiac CT can provide detailed images of the entire heart and surrounding vasculature. Multiplanar reformation and volume rendering of the data set allow three-dimensional reconstruction and visualization in any imaging plane. Compared with MRI, CT has a substantially shorter acquisition time, is more robust, has a higher spatial resolution, visualizes surrounding structures, and allows imaging of patients with metallic devices in place. These advantages come at the cost of a need for iodinated contrast agent and radiation.

After describing technical aspects, this article addresses the role of CT in radiofrequency ablation (particularly atrial fibrillation), cardiac resynchronization therapy, and then other electrophysiology-related conditions and procedures.

## TECHNIQUE OF CARDIAC CT FOR ELECTROPHYSIOLOGY APPLICATIONS

Despite having a very different purpose, the technique for performing cardiac CT for EP applications is very similar to that used for coronary imaging. The focus of CT for these applications is mainly structure and function. The duration of contrast administration and the timing of scan acquisition may vary slightly depending on the indication. As always, breath holding is crucial to minimize motion artifacts. Expiratory breath holding is preferred, as it allows more accurate coregistration with electroanatomical mapping data. Either retrospective electrocardiographic gating or prospective triggering is possible.[6] Prospective gating has the advantage of a very low radiation dosage; however, it is not as robust as retrospective gating unless the heart rate is slow and regular. In addition, because images are acquired in only one phase of the cardiac cycle, functional information, such as left ventricular (LV) ejection fraction, cannot be derived with prospective gating. If retrospective gating is being utilized, ECG-based tube current modulation should be used whenever possible. With either acquisition mode, one should consider lowering the peak kilovolt (eg, 100 kVp), especially in thinner patients. These measures will reduce the patient's

[a] Department of Radiology, Cardiac MR/CT Program, Cardiovascular Imaging Section, Massachusetts General Hospital, 165 Cambridge Street, Suite 400, Boston, MA 02114-2750, USA
[b] Department of Radiology, Section of Cardiology, Massachusetts General Hospital, 165 Cambridge Street, Suite 400, Boston, MA 02114-2750, USA
* Corresponding author.
*E-mail address:* sabbara@partners.org (S. Abbara).

Cardiol Clin 27 (2009) 619–631
doi:10.1016/j.ccl.2009.06.012
0733-8651/09/$ – see front matter 

radiation dose dramatically. For some patients electrocardiographic gating can be difficult. Because the duration of diastole varies with heart rate (cycle length of individual beats), systolic phases may provide better image quality in patients who have atrial fibrillation or frequent ectopy. The duration of systole is relatively constant for supraventricular beats, so image reconstruction at defined absolute time intervals (eg 150 and 250 milliseconds after the electrocardiographic QRS) is preferable to a percentage phase of the cardiac cycle. Scanners with high temporal resolution, such as those with dual-source or very rapid gantry rotation, are particularly helpful in overcoming motion artifacts related to arrhythmias.

## CT PRIOR TO RADIOFREQUENCY ABLATION

Radiofrequency ablation is an invasive catheter-based procedure that involves creating lesions to electrically isolate regions of the heart and so modify the substrate for arrhythmias.[4] Using venous femoral access, catheters are directed into cardiac chambers and sometimes across the interatrial septum. Typical targets for ablation include the isthmus between the inferior vena cava and tricuspid valve for atrial flutter ablation, the atrioventricular (AV) node, or accessory pathways from the atria to the ventricles for various forms of supraventricular tachycardia. CT can help define anatomy for these procedures, but by far the most common indication for CT is atrial fibrillation ablation. Atrial fibrillation often initiates from foci within sleeves of atrial tissue extending into the pulmonary veins.[7] Various ablation techniques have been devised to electrically isolate the pulmonary veins and interrupt the circuits that support the arrhythmia within the left atrium. Because of the anatomic variability and delicate nature of the pulmonary veins, imaging has become an essential part of the invasive management of atrial fibrillation.[8]

Prior to atrial fibrillation ablation, cardiac CT often is requested to aid in procedural planning. Given that opacification of the left atrium and pulmonary veins occurs only fractionally earlier than in the arterial circulation, the same duration of contrast administration and delay to image acquisition is used as for a coronary study. All vendors now offer software that allows for high-quality volume-rendered images of the left atrium. In addition to defining pulmonary venous anatomy, the volume of the left atrium can be measured accurately by CT, a parameter that predicts not only freedom from atrial fibrillation but also long-term cardiovascular morbidity.[9–11]

### *Pulmonary Vein Anatomy*

Typically, there are four pulmonary veins that enter into the left atrium by means of separate ostia. This normal arrangement is found in 56% of patients.[8] The anatomy can be visualized in simple axial images, but is depicted most vividly by three-dimensional volume rendering and by construction of an endoluminal view (**Fig. 1**). The diameters of each of the pulmonary veins then can be measured easily by manipulation of the data set to create a cross section of each pulmonary vein.

There are several well-recognized variants of pulmonary venous anatomy.[12,13] A common ostium of left pulmonary veins is found in 17% of patients, and is sometimes difficult to distinguish from separate openings.[8,12] A single ostium on the left side is larger than the most circular mapping

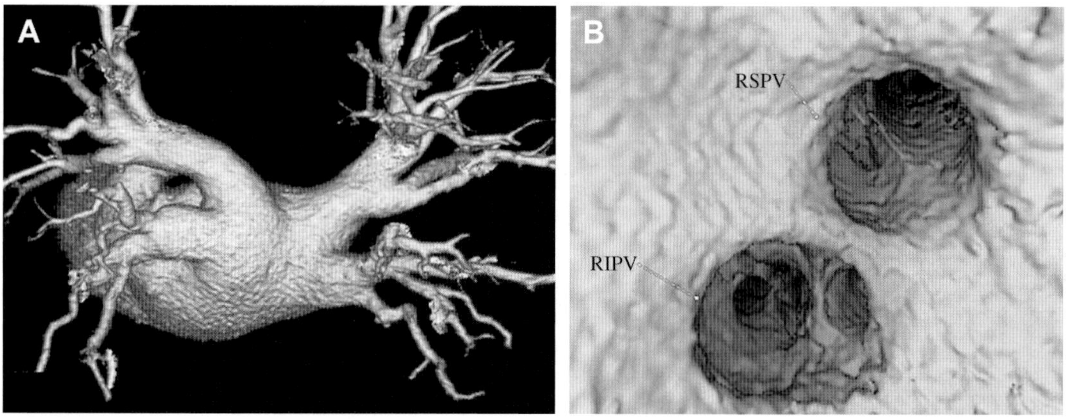


**Fig. 1.** (*A*) Three-dimensional volume-rendered CT image of posterior aspect of left atrium demonstrates normal pulmonary venous anatomy with four separate veins entering the left atrium. (*B*) Endoluminal view CT image of left atrium shows ostia of right inferior pulmonary vein (RIPV), and right superior pulmonary vein (RSPV).

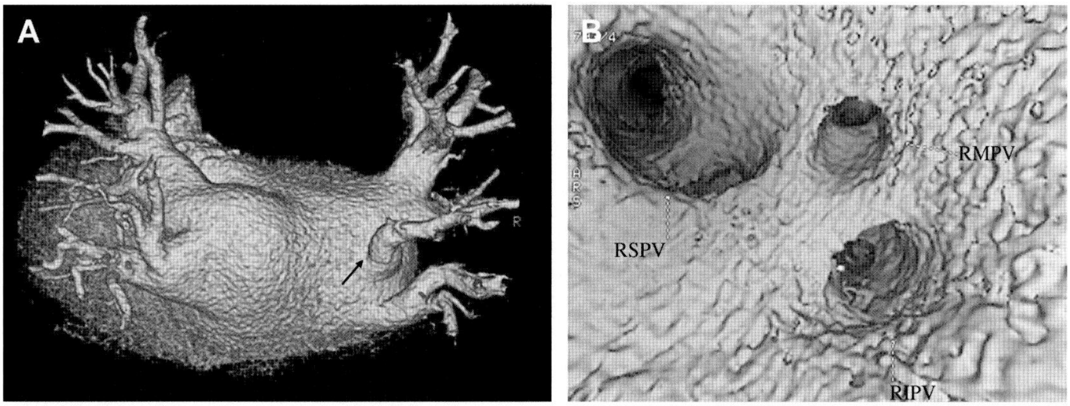


**Fig. 2.** (*A*) Three-dimensional volume-rendered CT image of posterior aspect of left atrium shows variant anatomy with a right middle pulmonary vein (*arrow*). (*B*) Endoluminal view CT image of left atrium shows three distinct right-sided pulmonary venous ostia. *Abbreviations:* RIPV, right inferior pulmonary vein RMPV, right middle pulmonary vein; RSPV = right superior pulmonary vein.

catheters; therefore segmental isolation is sometimes not possible in the presence of this variant.[5]

Accessory pulmonary veins are found in 29% of patients and can be of substantial clinical importance.[8,14] A right middle vein, draining the right middle lobe of the lung, is so common that it is considered a variant of normal (**Fig. 2**). If unrecognized, it is at risk of trauma during the ablation procedure and later of pulmonary vein stenosis. Modification of ablation technique may be required in the presence of a right middle vein, because a figure-of-eight ablation is not possible, and the rim of intervening tissue between veins may not be adequate to stably support the ablation catheter.[5] A top vein that drains into the superior aspect of the left atrium is less common but similarly at risk of trauma (**Fig. 3**).[15] Occasional rare variants include pulmonary veins that cross the midline posterior to the left atrium.[16] Such veins may be at risk not only from direct ablation at the venous ostia, but also during the application of radiofrequency energy to the posterior wall of the left atrium. Preprocedural CT also may uncover partial anomalous pulmonary venous return (PAPVR), a condition in which one or more pulmonary veins drain into the superior vena cava, right atrium, a left vertical vein, or the inferior vena cava (scimitar syndrome). PAPVR of the left upper lobe is essentially part of the spectrum of sinus venosus atrial septal defects, and its discovery should prompt thorough diagnostic investigation and reconsideration of the ablation procedure itself.

## *Esophageal Position*

Although usually requested to define pulmonary venous anatomy, other useful information can be obtained from CT performed prior to atrial fibrillation ablation. The relationship of the esophagus to the left atrium and pulmonary veins can be defined by cardiac CT.[17,18] The importance of this relationship lies in the risk of atrio–esophageal fistula, a rare but potentially lethal complication caused by radiofrequency burns extending into the esophagus through the left atrial or pulmonary venous wall.[19,20] To help recognize the esophagus during the ablation procedure, a small quantity of oral barium may be given to the patient just prior to CT acquisition (**Fig. 4**).[18] In 62% of patients, the esophagus lies immediately posterior to the left pulmonary veins, while in 15% of patients, it

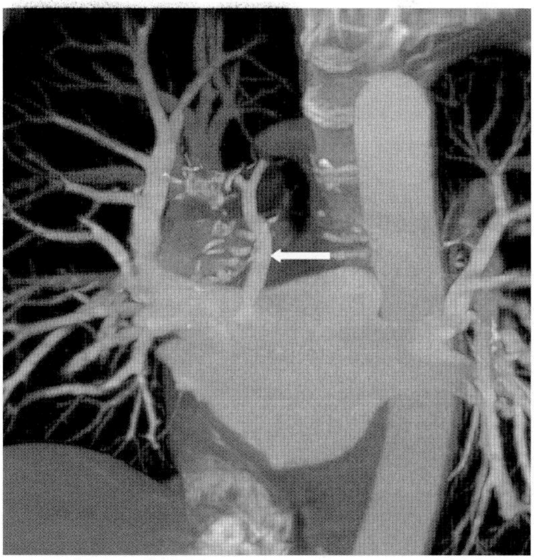

**Fig. 3.** Multiplanar reformatted thick maximum intensity projection CT image of left atrium in coronal projection shows a normal variant with an accessory vein (*right top vein, arrow*), which drains the lower lobe superior segment of the right lung.

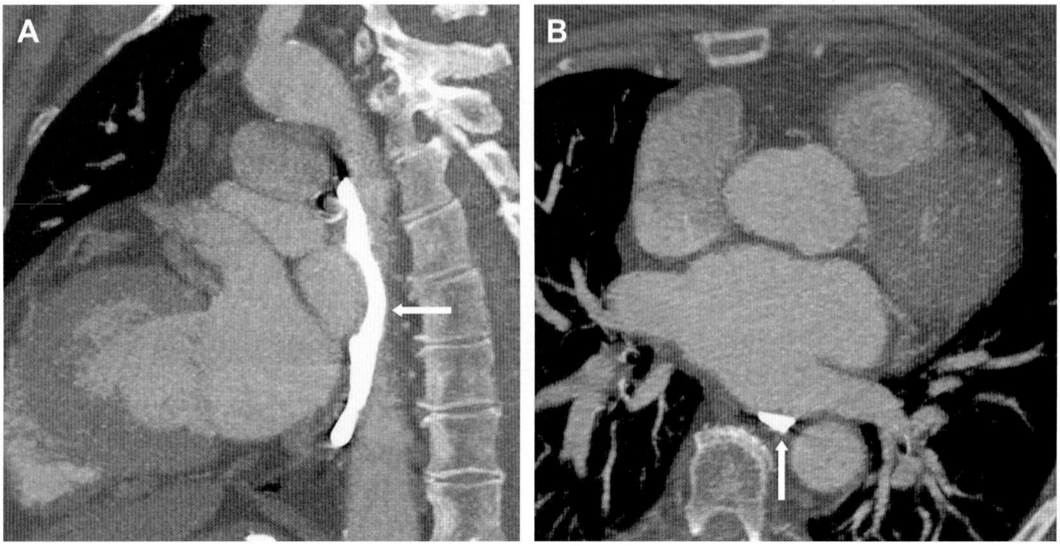

**Fig. 4.** Multiplanar reformatted CT images in oblique sagittal multiplanar reformation (*A*), and axial source image showing the location of the barium-filled esophagus (*arrows*) with respect to the left atrium and pulmonary veins (*B*). Although the esophageal location may be determined without barium use, its use permits coregistration of the esophagus during ablation procedures.

lies behind the right pulmonary veins (**Fig. 5**).[21] Lateral positioning of the esophagus relative to the heart can occur, however, and it remains unclear how accurately preprocedural CT predicts the anatomical relationship during ablation.[21,22]

## *Left Atrial Thrombi*

Thrombi also can be identified by CT as filling defects within the left atrial appendage.[23] Slow mixing of blood without thrombus, recognized as dense spontaneous echo contrast on ultrasound,

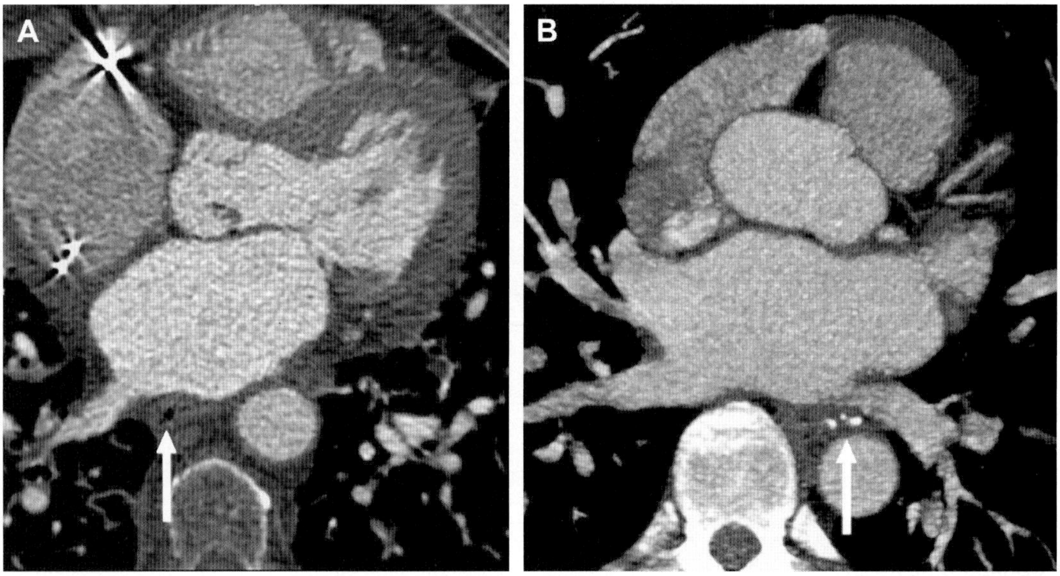

**Fig. 5.** Axial CT images in two different patients demonstrate the variability of esophageal location with respect to the pulmonary vein ostia. (*A*) The position of esophagus (*arrow*) is to the right of the midline and immediately adjacent to the right inferior pulmonary vein ostium. (*B*) Esophagus (*arrow*) is located to the left of the spine and adjacent to the left inferior pulmonary vein.

can give a similar appearance to thrombus on CT.[24] If in doubt, a delayed low-dose scan without additional contrast is performed after 1 minute to determine whether the filling defect persists (**Figs. 6** and **7**). CT is highly sensitive for detection of left atrial appendage thrombi but in absence of a delayed scan lacks specificity[25]; transesophageal echocardiography is recommended to confirm positive findings.

### *Procedural Guidance*

Integration of CT (or MRI) images and electroanatomic mapping has been a major advance in electrophysiology (**Fig. 8**).[26,27] A CT dataset that was acquired prior to the procedure can be coregistered with an electrical map created in the procedure laboratory to allow real-time guidance of the EP catheter.[28] Coregistration may be more difficult in patients who have marked left atrial enlargement, but perhaps surprisingly, the cardiac rhythm during CT acquisition does not seem to hinder image integration greatly (**Fig. 9**).[29,30] The hope is that CT image integration will reduce fluoroscopy time, improve procedural success, and reduce the recurrence of atrial fibrillation; however, the evidence is not conclusive.[31,32] In institutions where it is readily available, CT image integration has been become a standard part atrial fibrillation ablation. More exciting still is the development of remote navigation.[33,34] CT image integration and magnetic control of catheters allow the procedure to be performed at a distance, thus reducing radiation exposure for the operator. Remote catheter navigation also may prove to be more effective than the traditional technique for manipulating catheters into position.

## EVALUATION AFTER CATHETER ABLATION

CT also has a role after atrial fibrillation procedures. A well-recognized complication of atrial fibrillation ablation is pulmonary vein stenosis.[35] This complication usually presents within a year after the ablation procedure with dyspnea and other findings sometimes reminiscent of pulmonary embolus. Although relatively easy to suspect clinically, CT, MRI, or trans-esophageal echocardiography is required to confirm the diagnosis. By CT, stenosis is easy to identify, particularly if CT was used before the procedure and is available for comparison (**Fig. 10**). Unlike in MRI, where metallic stents lead to substantial artifact and signal drop-out, the large stents used to treat pulmonary vein stenosis are easy to interrogate for restenosis on CT. With the reduction in frequency of this complication, routine postprocedure imaging for pulmonary vein stenosis no longer is performed.[5]

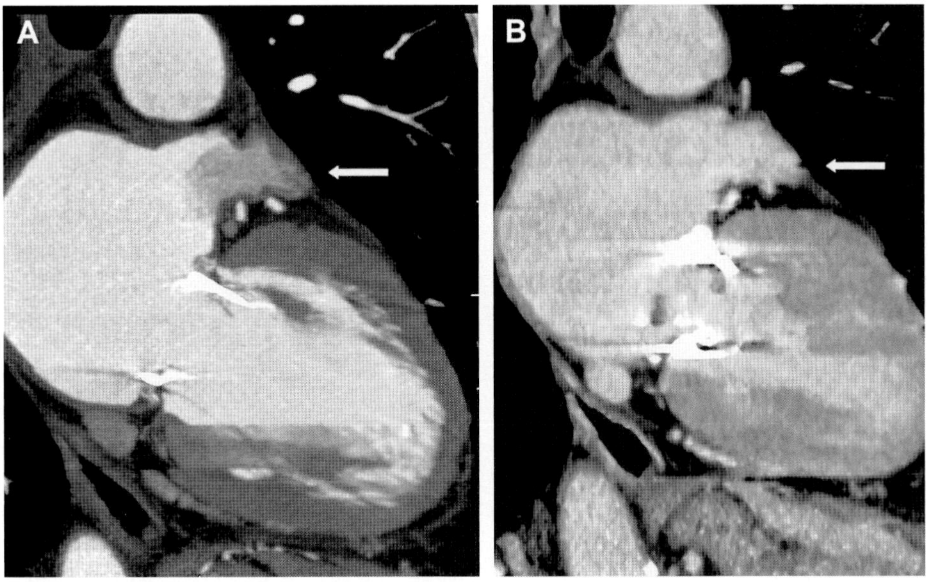


**Fig. 6.** Two-chamber view multiplanar reformatted CT images in the same patient in arterial phase (*A*) and a 1-minute delayed phase (*B*) show a filling defect in left atrial appendage on the early arterial phase, but on the phase acquired 1 minute later without further contrast administration, there is complete filling in of the atrial appendage, indicating absence of thrombus. (*From* Abbara S, Walker TG. Diagnostic imaging—cardiovascular. Salt Lake City (UT): Amirsys Incorporated; 2008. ISBN 978-1-4160-3340-0; with permission.)

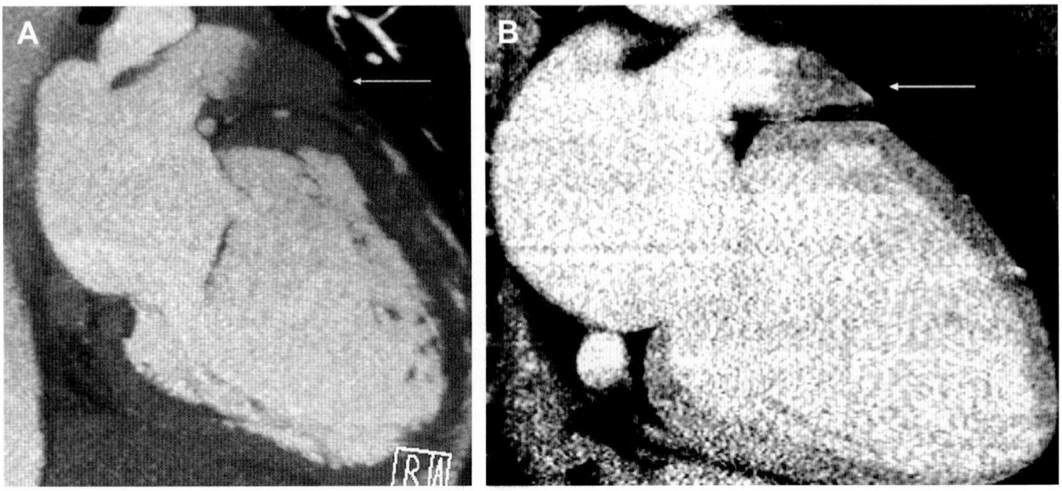


**Fig. 7.** Two-chamber view multiplanar reformatted CT image in the same patient in arterial phase (*A*) and a 1-minute delayed phase (*B*) shows a filling defect within the left atrial appendage (*arrow*) on the arterial phase, and a persistent filling defect on the delayed phase acquired at 1 minute, indicating presence of thrombus.

## USE OF CT FOR OTHER ELECTROPHYSIOLOGY PROCEDURES

Although atrial fibrillation is the main clinical indication for which cardiac CT is requested, there are potential uses for CT with other ablation procedures. As targets for ablation become increasing obscure and difficult to navigate, CT may be useful to define specific parts of cardiac anatomy. The aortic cusps, the coronary sinus, and many other locations within the atria have been identified as foci for tachycardia and thus potential targets for ablation.[36–38] Long considered beyond the reach of the catheter, mapping and ablation at the epicardium now are being performed.[39] CT can be used to define the extent and distribution of epicardial fat,[40] a factor that may influence the feasibility and success of epicardial ablation and

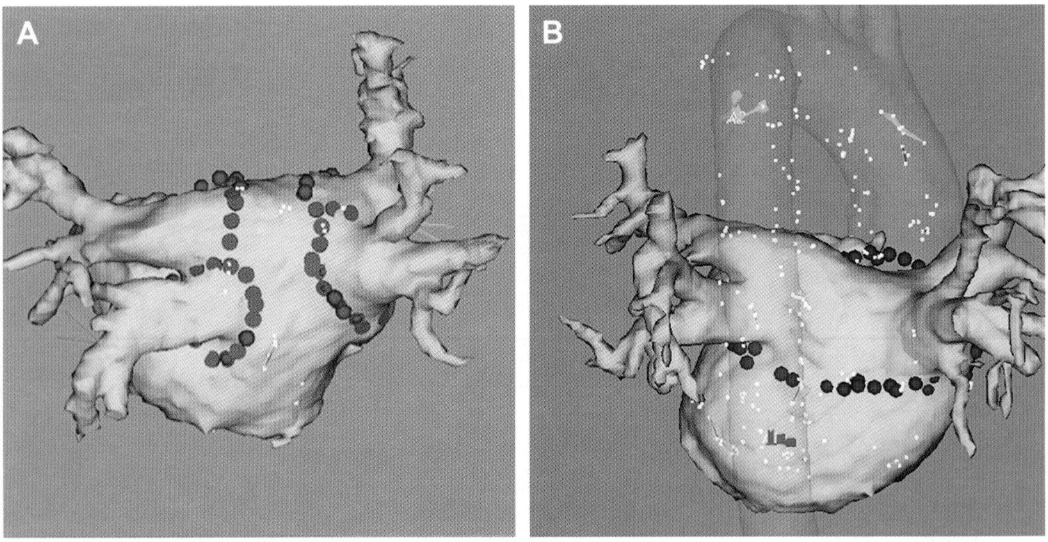


**Fig. 8.** (*A*) Volume-rendered CT image integrated into electro-anatomic map during radiofrequency ablation showing separate isolation of all pulmonary veins with four separate circles. The small white dots indicate anatomical reference points that are obtained by means of catheter tip coordinate localization during the procedure (anatomic mapping), and the red and grey dots indicate radiofrequency ablation points. (*B*) Volume-rendered CT image integrated into electro-anatomic map during radiofrequency ablation shows good coregistration with aorta and isolation of all four pulmonary veins with one circle.

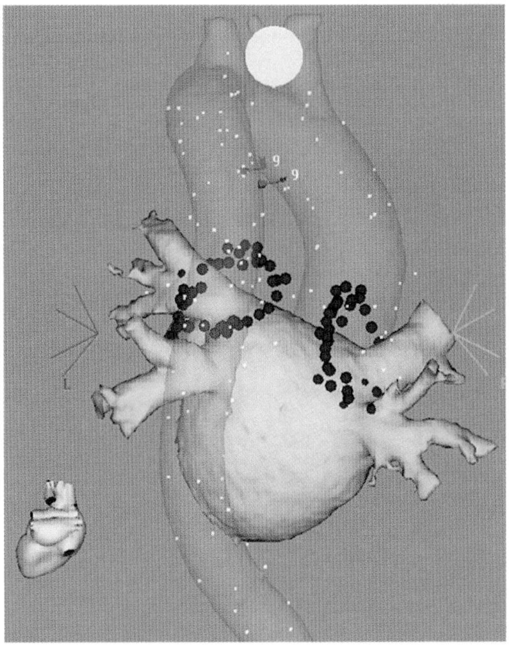

**Fig. 9.** Volume-rendered CT image incorporated into electro-anatomic map shows poor coregistration of data caused by CT acquisition during inspiration rather than expiration.

map the coronary artery course. Although delayed hyperenhancement imaging by CT remains inferior to MRI, the potential exists for CT to define the extent of scar within the heart caused by previous myocardial infarction or ablation and thus guide subsequent therapy.

## CT IN CARDIAC RESYNCHRONIZATION THERAPY

Cardiac resynchronization therapy (CRT) is a treatment for advanced heart failure that involves placing a lead within the coronary venous system to pace the left ventricle.[41] The aim is to restore the coordination of the left ventricle by correcting differences in the timing of contraction (dyssynchrony). CRT has proven to be remarkably effective in improving symptoms and also in prolonging life in certain subgroups of patients who have heart failure.[1]

Implantation of the pacing lead within the coronary venous system can be challenging. A venogram usually is performed in the cardiac catheterization laboratory during the procedure, but the information derived is limited by its two-dimensional nature, although rotational venography is a promising tool that may help overcome this limitation. The coronary venous anatomy can be defined preprocedurally by cardiac CT (**Fig. 11**).[42,43] The image acquisition is similar to that for coronary imaging, other than that the delay to imaging after contrast administration is greater to allow capture of the venous phase of enhancement. Based on the CT image, a target vein can be identified, ideally one that corresponds with the myocardial segment with most delayed contraction.

Coronary venous anatomy varies considerably between patients.[44,45] The great cardiac vein and middle cardiac vein, running in the anterior and inferior interventricular grooves respectively, are present in almost all patients.[43] The target veins

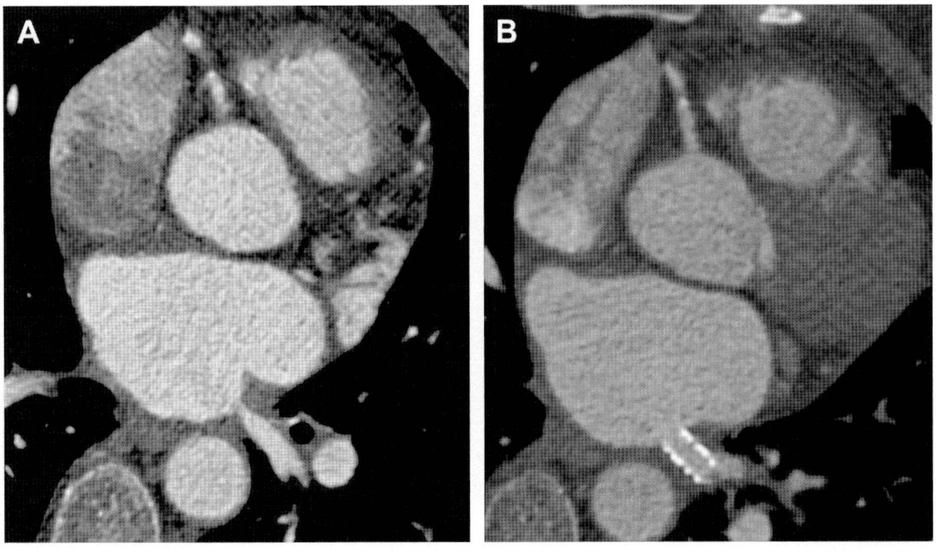


**Fig. 10.** Axial CT images of same patient prior to (*A*) and after (*B*) percutaneous intervention. (*A*) Ostial left inferior pulmonary vein stenosis in a patient who had previous radiofrequency ablation for atrial fibrillation. (*B*) Postintervention CT after stent implantation shows patent left inferior pulmonary vein stent without evidence of restenosis.

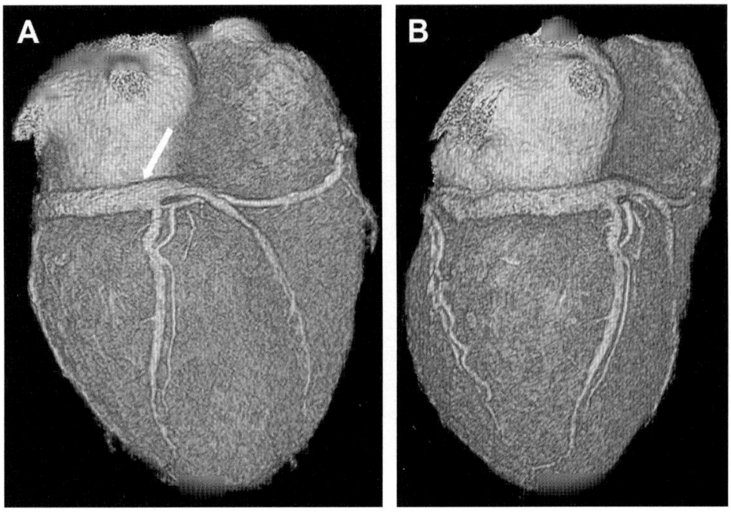


**Fig. 11.** Volume-rendered CT images optimized to demonstrate coronary venous anatomy prior to implantation of biventricular pacemaker. (*A*) Inferior or diaphragmatic view shows coronary sinus (*arrow*), middle cardiac vein, and a marginal vein. The lateral view (*B*) shows the great cardiac vein running in the left atrioventricular groove.

for CRT, the lateral or posterior cardiac veins, show substantial variability, however, and in 1% to 3% of patients, they are absent.[43] In particular, the lateral cardiac vein is usually absent in patients who have prior lateral myocardial infarction.[46] Thebesian valves, located at the opening of the coronary sinus into the left atrium, are of importance, as they may hinder passage of the pacing lead into the left ventricle. In approximately one third of patients, some remnant of a Thebesian valve can be identified.[47] Although CT has yet to be shown to improve CRT procedural success or efficiency, the marked variability in coronary venous anatomy makes anatomical information desirable.

A recent exciting development is the use of CT to assess dyssynchrony.[48] Although yet to be shown predictive of response to CRT, the ability to assess coronary venous anatomy, LV function, and dyssynchrony make CT a valuable tool prior to CRT.

## OTHER INDICATIONS

Atrial appendage occluders, such as the Watchman device (Atritech Inc., Plymouth, Minnesota), are used to prevent thrombus formation and reduce the risk of stroke.[49] CT can be used preprocedurally to define appendage morphology and after the procedure to confirm that the appendage has been excluded from the circulation (**Figs. 12–14**).[50] Similarly, CT can be used to image other intracardiac devices such as pacemakers and defibrillators. Pacing lead position occasionally can be difficult to ascertain by other techniques, and CT may be helpful in diagnosing right ventricular (RV) perforation or other forms of malposition.

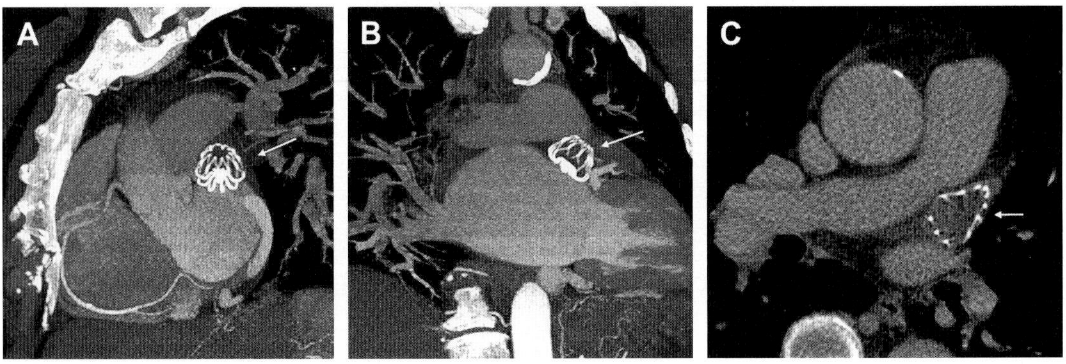


**Fig. 12.** Multiplanar reformatted thick maximum-intensity projection CT images (*A, B*) and an axial source image (*C*) show a Watchman occluder device (Atritech Inc., Plymouth, Minnesota) in left atrial appendage (*arrow*). Note absence of contrast material within the excluded atrial appendage.

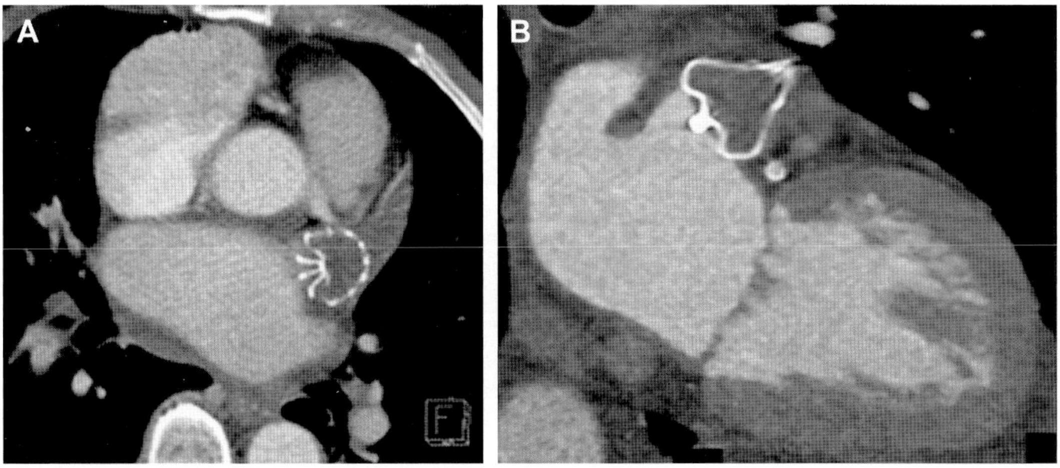


**Fig. 13.** Axial oblique (*A*) and two-chamber long axis (*B*) multiplanar reformatted views of cardiac CT show Watchman device successfully occluding left atrial appendage, as evidenced by the absence of contrast within the excluded appendage.

There are several other situations in which CT may be helpful to the electrophysiologist. Not infrequently MRI would be preferable but may be contraindicated because of the presence of a pacemaker or other ferromagnetic device.

LV ejection fraction can be measured by retrospectively gated cardiac CT.[51,52] Ejection fraction calculations are possible even if tube current modulation is used, and tube-current modulation should be used (with only rare exceptions) to minimize radiation dose. Theoretically, CT may underestimate LV ejection fraction slightly by missing the time of minimum end systolic volume. This potential slight systematic error is of no clinical consequence other than when using strict ejection fraction criteria for device eligibility.[53] CT also has been used for the diagnosis of arrhythmogenic RV dysplasia (ARVD).[54] ARVD is diagnosed by using a set of major and minor criteria. Presence of two major, or one major and two minor, or four minor criteria establishes the diagnosis. CT has the potential to identify presence of major or miner criteria for ARVD, including focal or global RV dysfunction and localized aneurysm formation.[55,56] Intramyocardial fat, a major criterion if

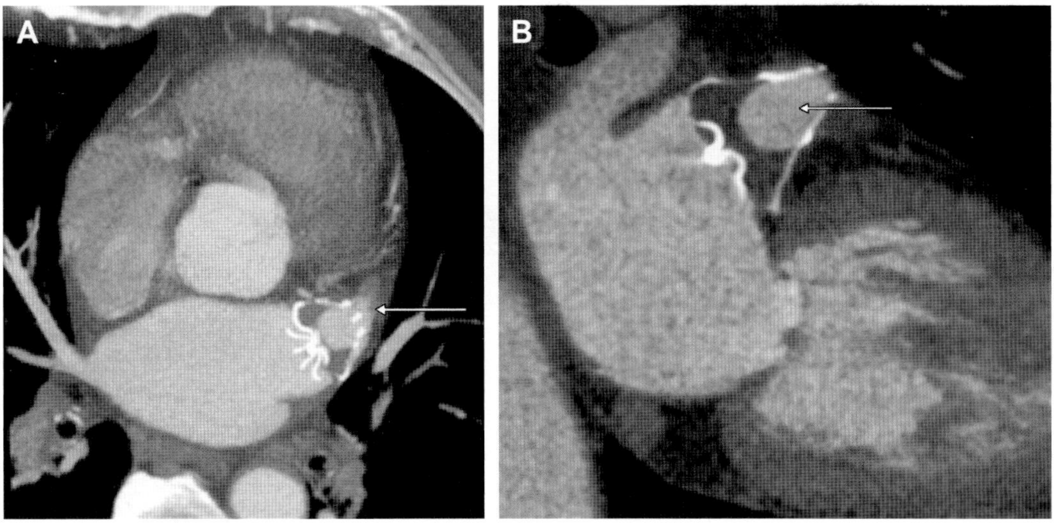


**Fig. 14.** Axial oblique (*A*) and two-chamber long axis (*B*) multiplanar reformatted views of cardiac CT show Watchman device with incomplete occlusion of left atrial appendage indicated by presence of contrast within the appendage (*arrows*).

detected on pathology, sometimes can be recognized as an area of low attenuation within the RV wall.[57] The incidental detection of intramyocardial RV fat by CT is relatively common and of uncertain clinical significance, however. Increased trabeculation and scalloping of the RV wall are also more common in patients who have ARVD compared with controls; however, firm diagnostic criteria have not been established.[54] In general, CT is helpful, mainly in establishing that RV function and morphology are clearly normal, or by identifying gross abnormalities in the right ventricle such as RV aneurysms or global dysfunction.

## FUTURE DIRECTIONS

Rapid advances in hardware and software will lead to broader indications for cardiac CT. Of particular relevance to EP are the improvements in temporal resolution brought about by faster gantry rotation speeds and dual-source imaging. Improved temporal resolution means fewer motion artifacts and higher image quality in patients who have irregular and fast heart rates.[58] With increasing numbers of detector rows, the largest now being 320 detectors, the overall scan time is being reduced such that the ability to sustain a prolonged breath hold is no longer necessary. Software is improving rapidly and promises to allow increasingly rapid automated postprocessing.

An important area of progress in cardiac CT relates to reducing radiation exposure. Radiation dose is cumulative, and the lifetime risk of malignancy is highly dependent on age.[59] The ALARA (as low as reasonably achievable) always should be adhered to in cardiac CT; however, the radiation dose delivered with most scan protocols remains substantial. Prospective triggering dramatically reduces radiation dose by imaging only for a small fraction of the cardiac cycle.[60] Although repeated cardiac CT scanning is not recommended, the two decades or so required for malignancy to develop makes radiation less of an issue in the elderly and others with life expectancy limited by serious medical conditions.

Perhaps the greatest challenge, although yet to be recognized fully, is the burden of proof regarding the value and cost-effectiveness of cardiac imaging.[61] The ability to obtain exquisite pictures may not be sufficient justification for the routine use of CT prior to EP procedures; tangible benefits need to be demonstrated. Appropriateness criteria for cardiac imaging are a step forward in this regard, and clinical trials assessing a strategy of imaging prior to a procedure are awaited.[62]

## SUMMARY

Not only are rapid advances in cardiac CT helping to facilitate progress in EP, but new EP techniques are helping drive development in CT. Cardiac CT is becoming an integral part of arrhythmia management to define pulmonary vein anatomy before ablation, to facilitate electroanatomic mapping during the procedure with CT image integration, and to diagnose potential complications such as pulmonary vein stenosis. CT has an emerging role in cardiac resynchronization therapy in defining cardiac venous anatomy, and potentially in patient selection through LV functional and dyssynchrony assessment. Whenever detailed three-dimensional images of the heart and vasculature are required, CT is an ideal imaging modality. As accessibility to CT grows, so will the breadth of applications relevant to electrophysiology.

## REFERENCES


1. Cleland JG, Daubert JC, Erdmann E, et al. The effect of cardiac resynchronization on morbidity and mortality in heart failure. N Engl J Med 2005; 352(15):1539–49.
2. Bristow MR, Saxon LA, Boehmer J, et al. Cardiac resynchronization therapy with or without an implantable defibrillator in advanced chronic heart failure. N Engl J Med 2004;350(21):2140–50.
3. Hunt SA, Abraham WT, Chin MH, et al. ACC/AHA 2005 guideline update for the diagnosis and management of chronic heart failure in the adult: a report of the American College of Cardiology/ American Heart Association Task Force on Practice Guidelines (Writing Committee to Update the 2001 Guidelines for the Evaluation and Management of Heart Failure). Developed in collaboration with the American College of Chest Physicians and the International Society for Heart and Lung Transplantation: endorsed by the Heart Rhythm Society. Circulation 2005;112(12):e154–235.
4. Morady F. Radiofrequency ablation as treatment for cardiac arrhythmias. N Engl J Med 1999;340(7): 534–44.
5. Mansour M, Holmvang G, Ruskin J. Role of imaging techniques in preparation for catheter ablation of atrial fibrillation. J Cardiovasc Electrophysiol 2004; 15(9):1107–8.
6. Moloo J, Shapiro MD, Abbara S. Cardiac computed tomography: technique and optimization of protocols. Semin Roentgenol 2008;43(2):90–9.
7. Haissaguerre M, Jais P, Shah DC, et al. Spontaneous initiation of atrial fibrillation by ectopic beats originating in the pulmonary veins. N Engl J Med 1998;339(10):659–66.

8. Mansour M, Holmvang G, Sosnovik D, et al. Assessment of pulmonary vein anatomic variability by magnetic resonance imaging: implications for catheter ablation techniques for atrial fibrillation. J Cardiovasc Electrophysiol 2004;15(4):387–93.
9. Shin SH, Park MY, Oh WJ, et al. Left atrial volume is a predictor of atrial fibrillation recurrence after catheter ablation. J Am Soc Echocardiogr 2008;21(6): 697–702.
10. Gerdts E, Wachtell K, Omvik P, et al. Left atrial size and risk of major cardiovascular events during antihypertensive treatment: losartan intervention for endpoint reduction in hypertension trial. Hypertension 2007;49(2):311–6.
11. Osranek M, Bursi F, Bailey KR, et al. Left atrial volume predicts cardiovascular events in patients originally diagnosed with lone atrial fibrillation: three-decade follow-up. Eur Heart J 2005;26(23):2556–61.
12. Ahmed J, Sohal S, Malchano ZJ, et al. Three-dimensional analysis of pulmonary venous ostial and antral anatomy: implications for balloon catheter-based pulmonary vein isolation. J Cardiovasc Electrophysiol 2006;17(3):251–5.
13. Kaseno K, Tada H, Koyama K, et al. Prevalence and characterization of pulmonary vein variants in patients with atrial fibrillation determined using 3-dimensional computed tomography. Am J Cardiol 2008;101(11):1638–42.
14. Mansour M, Holmvang G, Mela T, et al. Anterior and posterior right middle pulmonary veins in a patient undergoing catheter ablation for atrial fibrillation [case report]. J Cardiovasc Electrophysiol 2004; 15(10):1231.
15. Arslan G, Dincer E, Kabaalioglu A, et al. Right top pulmonary vein: evaluation with 64 section multidetector computed tomography. Eur J Radiol 2008; 67(2):300–3.
16. Sarwar A, Nasir K, Shapiro MD, et al. Anomalous left inferior pulmonary vein crossing midline and draining via common ostium with right inferior pulmonary vein [case report]. J Cardiovasc Electrophysiol 2008;19(2):223.
17. Tsao HM, Wu MH, Higa S, et al. Anatomic relationship of the esophagus and left atrium: implication for catheter ablation of atrial fibrillation. Chest 2005;128(4):2581–7.
18. Cury RC, Abbara S, Schmidt S, et al. Relationship of the esophagus and aorta to the left atrium and pulmonary veins: implications for catheter ablation of atrial fibrillation. Heart Rhythm 2005;2(12): 1317–23.
19. Cummings JE, Schweikert RA, Saliba WI, et al. Brief communication: atrial–esophageal fistulas after radiofrequency ablation. Ann Intern Med 2006; 144(8):572–4.
20. Pappone C, Oral H, Santinelli V, et al. Atrio–esophageal fistula as a complication of percutaneous transcatheter ablation of atrial fibrillation. Circulation 2004;109(22):2724–6.
21. Daoud EG, Hummel JD, Houmsse M, et al. Comparison of computed tomography imaging with intraprocedural contrast esophagram: implications for catheter ablation of atrial fibrillation. Heart Rhythm 2008;5(7):975–80.
22. Piorkowski C, Hindricks G, Schreiber D, et al. Electroanatomic reconstruction of the left atrium, pulmonary veins, and esophagus compared with the true anatomy on multislice computed tomography in patients undergoing catheter ablation of atrial fibrillation. Heart Rhythm 2006;3(3):317–27.
23. Kim YY, Klein AL, Halliburton SS, et al. Left atrial appendage filling defects identified by multidetector computed tomography in patients undergoing radiofrequency pulmonary vein antral isolation: a comparison with transesophageal echocardiography. Am Heart J 2007;154(6):1199–205.
24. Shapiro MD, Neilan TG, Jassal DS, et al. Multidetector computed tomography for the detection of left atrial appendage thrombus: a comparative study with transesophageal echocardiography. J Comput Assist Tomogr 2007;31(6):905–9.
25. Patel A, Au E, Donegan K, et al. Multidetector row computed tomography for identification of left atrial appendage filling defects in patients undergoing pulmonary vein isolation for treatment of atrial fibrillation: comparison with transesophageal echocardiography. Heart Rhythm 2008;5(2):253–60.
26. Malchano ZJ, Neuzil P, Cury RC, et al. Integration of cardiac CT/MR imaging with three-dimensional electroanatomical mapping to guide catheter manipulation in the left atrium: implications for catheter ablation of atrial fibrillation. J Cardiovasc Electrophysiol 2006;17(11):1221–9.
27. Tops LF, Bax JJ, Zeppenfeld K, et al. Fusion of multislice computed tomography imaging with three-dimensional electroanatomic mapping to guide radiofrequency catheter ablation procedures. Heart Rhythm 2005;2(10):1076–81.
28. Kistler PM, Earley MJ, Harris S, et al. Validation of three-dimensional cardiac image integration: use of integrated CT image into electroanatomic mapping system to perform catheter ablation of atrial fibrillation. J Cardiovasc Electrophysiol 2006;17(4):341–8.
29. Heist EK, Chevalier J, Holmvang G, et al. Factors affecting error in integration of electroanatomic mapping with CT and MR imaging during catheter ablation of atrial fibrillation. J Interv Card Electrophysiol 2006;17(1):21–7.
30. Patel AM, Heist EK, Chevalier J, et al. Effect of presenting rhythm on image integration to direct catheter ablation of atrial fibrillation. J Interv Card Electrophysiol 2008;22(3):205–10.
31. Kistler PM, Rajappan K, Jahngir M, et al. The impact of CT image integration into an electroanatomic

mapping system on clinical outcomes of catheter ablation of atrial fibrillation. J Cardiovasc Electrophysiol 2006;17(10):1093–101.
32. Kistler PM, Rajappan K, Harris S, et al. The impact of image integration on catheter ablation of atrial fibrillation using electroanatomic mapping: a prospective randomized study. Eur Heart J 2008;29(24):3029–36.
33. Aryana A, d'Avila A, Heist EK, et al. Remote magnetic navigation to guide endocardial and epicardial catheter mapping of scar-related ventricular tachycardia. Circulation 2007;115(10):1191–200.
34. Reddy VY, Neuzil P, Malchano ZJ, et al. View-synchronized robotic image-guided therapy for atrial fibrillation ablation: experimental validation and clinical feasibility. Circulation 2007;115(21):2705–14.
35. Saad EB, Marrouche NF, Saad CP, et al. Pulmonary vein stenosis after catheter ablation of atrial fibrillation: emergence of a new clinical syndrome. Ann Intern Med 2003;138(8):634–8.
36. Das S, Neuzil P, Albert CM, et al. Catheter ablation of peri-AV nodal atrial tachycardia from the noncoronary cusp of the aortic valve. J Cardiovasc Electrophysiol 2008;19(3):231–7.
37. Kistler PM, Fynn SP, Haqqani H, et al. Focal atrial tachycardia from the ostium of the coronary sinus: electrocardiographic and electrophysiological characterization and radiofrequency ablation. J Am Coll Cardiol 2005;45(9):1488–93.
38. Kistler PM, Roberts-Thomson KC, Haqqani HM, et al. P-wave morphology in focal atrial tachycardia: development of an algorithm to predict the anatomic site of origin. J Am Coll Cardiol 2006;48(5):1010–7.
39. Sosa E, Scanavacca M. Epicardial mapping and ablation techniques to control ventricular tachycardia. J Cardiovasc Electrophysiol 2005;16(4):449–52.
40. Abbara S, Desai JC, Cury RC, et al. Mapping epicardial fat with multidetector computed tomography to facilitate percutaneous transepicardial arrhythmia ablation. Eur J Radiol 2006;57(3):417–22.
41. Jarcho JA. Resynchronizing ventricular contraction in heart failure. N Engl J Med 2005;352(15):1594–7.
42. Muhlenbruch G, Koos R, Wildberger JE, et al. Imaging of the cardiac venous system: comparison of MDCT and conventional angiography. AJR Am J Roentgenol 2005;185(5):1252–7.
43. Abbara S, Cury RC, Nieman K, et al. Noninvasive evaluation of cardiac veins with 16-MDCT angiography. AJR Am J Roentgenol 2005;185(4):1001–6.
44. Jongbloed MR, Lamb HJ, Bax JJ, et al. Noninvasive visualization of the cardiac venous system using multislice computed tomography. J Am Coll Cardiol 2005;45(5):749–53.
45. Blendea D, Shah RV, Auricchio A, et al. Variability of coronary venous anatomy in patients undergoing cardiac resynchronization therapy: a high-speed rotational venography study. Heart Rhythm 2007;4(9):1155–62.
46. Van de Veire NR, Schuijf JD, De Sutter J, et al. Noninvasive visualization of the cardiac venous system in coronary artery disease patients using 64-slice computed tomography. J Am Coll Cardiol 2006;48(9):1832–8.
47. Christiaens L, Ardilouze P, Ragot S, et al. Prospective evaluation of the anatomy of the coronary venous system using multidetector row computed tomography. Int J Cardiol 2008;126(2):204–8.
48. Truong QA, Singh JP, Cannon CP, et al. Quantitative analysis of intraventricular dyssynchrony using wall thickness by multidetector computed tomography. JACC Cardiovasc Imaging 2008;1:772–81.
49. Sick PB, Schuler G, Hauptmann KE, et al. Initial worldwide experience with the WATCHMAN left atrial appendage system for stroke prevention in atrial fibrillation. J Am Coll Cardiol 2007;49(13):1490–5.
50. Heist EK, Refaat M, Danik SB, et al. Analysis of the left atrial appendage by magnetic resonance angiography in patients with atrial fibrillation. Heart Rhythm 2006;3(11):1313–8.
51. Schlosser T, Mohrs OK, Magedanz A, et al. Assessment of left ventricular function and mass in patients undergoing computed tomography (CT) coronary angiography using 64-detector row CT: comparison to magnetic resonance imaging. Acta Radiol 2007;48(1):30–5.
52. Raman SV, Shah M, McCarthy B, et al. Multi-detector row cardiac computed tomography accurately quantifies right and left ventricular size and function compared with cardiac magnetic resonance. Am Heart J 2006;151(3):736–44.
53. Moss AJ, Zareba W, Hall WJ, et al. Prophylactic implantation of a defibrillator in patients with myocardial infarction and reduced ejection fraction. N Engl J Med 2002;346(12):877–83.
54. Bomma C, Dalal D, Tandri H, et al. Evolving role of multidetector computed tomography in evaluation of arrhythmogenic right ventricular dysplasia/cardiomyopathy. Am J Cardiol 2007;100(1):99–105.
55. Tandri H, Macedo R, Calkins H, et al. Role of magnetic resonance imaging in arrhythmogenic right ventricular dysplasia: insights from the North American arrhythmogenic right ventricular dysplasia (ARVD/C) study. Am Heart J 2008;155(1):147–53.
56. McKenna WJ, Thiene G, Nava A, et al. Diagnosis of arrhythmogenic right ventricular dysplasia/cardiomyopathy. Task Force of the Working Group Myocardial and Pericardial Disease of the European Society of Cardiology and of the Scientific Council on Cardiomyopathies of the International Society and Federation of Cardiology. Br Heart J 1994;71(3):215–8.

57. Raney AR, Saremi F, Kenchaiah S, et al. Multidetector computed tomography shows intramyocardial fat deposition. J Cardiovasc Comput Tomogr 2008;2(3): 152–63.
58. Matt D, Scheffel H, Leschka S, et al. Dual-source CT coronary angiography: image quality, mean heart rate, and heart rate variability. AJR Am J Roentgenol 2007;189(3):567–73.
59. Einstein AJ, Henzlova MJ, Rajagopalan S. Estimating risk of cancer associated with radiation exposure from 64-slice computed tomography coronary angiography. JAMA 2007;298(3):317–23.
60. Husmann L, Valenta I, Gaemperli O, et al. Feasibility of low-dose coronary CT angiography: first experience with prospective ECG gating. Eur Heart J 2008;29(2):191–7.
61. Gibbons RJ. Leading the elephant out of the corner: the future of health care: presidential address at the American Heart Association 2006 scientific sessions. Circulation 2007;115(16): 2221–30.
62. Hendel RC, Patel MR, Kramer CM, et al. ACCF/ACR/SCCT/SCMR/ASNC/NASCI/SCAI/SIR 2006 appropriateness criteria for cardiac computed tomography and cardiac magnetic resonance imaging: a report of the American College of Cardiology Foundation Quality Strategic Directions Committee Appropriateness Criteria Working Group, American College of Radiology, Society of Cardiovascular Computed Tomography, Society for Cardiovascular Magnetic Resonance, American Society of Nuclear Cardiology, North American Society for Cardiac Imaging, Society for Cardiovascular Angiography and Interventions, and Society of Interventional Radiology. J Am Coll Cardiol 2006;48(7):1475–97.

# Evaluation of Cardiac Valves Using Multidetector CT

Juan Gaztanaga, MD, Gonzalo Pizarro, MD, Javier Sanz, MD*

**KEYWORDS**

- Computed tomography • Valves • Multidetector
- Aortic • Mitral

Recent technological advances in multidetector computed tomography (MDCT) scanners have allowed lower radiation dose and higher spatial and temporal resolutions, making fast heart rates and arrhythmias less of a limiting factor. This improvement has increased the number of potential applications of cardiac CT, although most patients still are referred for coronary CT angiography (CTA). During a routine CT of the heart, all four cardiac valves are imaged and may be visualized. Valvular calcification, particularly of left heart valves, is a frequent incidental finding on chest and cardiac CT scans and can be seen in up to 30% of patients.[1–3] In addition to the detection of valvular calcium, ECG gating has enabled the evaluation of leaflet morphology and function during a contrast-enhanced CTA, even in the absence of calcification.

The frequent identification of valve calcium on CT illustrates the prevalence of valvular heart disease (VHD), which affects 2.5% of all adults in the United States. The left-sided valves are involved more frequently, and mitral regurgitation (MR) is the leading cause of VHD.[4] In general, the initial clinical sign observed in VHD is a murmur during a physical examination. Occasionally, the first indication of VHD is the presence of symptoms from cardiac remodeling and/or hemodynamic compromise. The initial and preferred diagnostic test is Doppler transthoracic echocardiography.[5] Its high resolution, excellent safety profile, and visualization of both valvular anatomy and blood flow makes echocardiography the current cornerstone of VHD evaluation. Cardiac catheterization, long regarded as the reference test for the hemodynamic significance of valvular abnormalities, is performed less commonly now, although it still may be needed when the results of noninvasive tests are inconclusive. Moreover, invasive coronary angiography (CA) frequently is necessary to rule out significant coronary artery disease (CAD) preoperatively if surgical correction is indicated. Cardiac magnetic resonance has emerged as the most robust noninvasive alternative to echocardiography for VHD evaluation. Magnetic resonance usually is reserved for patients who have poor acoustic windows, inconclusive noninvasive results, discrepancies between echocardiography and catheterization, or a mismatch between diagnostic testing and symptoms. Cardiac CT for VHD assessment might be considered under the same circumstances, although CT has the disadvantages of depicting anatomy but not flow and of requiring ionizing radiation and nephrotoxic contrast agents. Therefore, it is unlikely that a cardiac CT will be performed exclusively for valvular evaluation unless the echocardiography is insufficient and there are contraindications for magnetic resonance (ie, the presence of a defibrillator). Useful information regarding valvular status or even calcium scoring can be obtained during a conventional coronary CTA, however. Moreover, growing evidence supports the use of coronary CTA to rule out significant CAD before valvular surgery in selected patients. This article reviews the most common CT findings associated with VHD and discusses technical aspects for optimal valvular assessment.

Dr. Sanz has served as a consultant for G.E. Healthcare.
Division of Cardiology, Department of Medicine, Mount Sinai School of Medicine, One Gustave Levy Place, Box 1030, New York, NY 10029, USA
* Corresponding author.
*E-mail address:* Javier.Sanz@mssm.edu (J. Sanz).

Cardiol Clin 27 (2009) 633–644
doi:10.1016/j.ccl.2009.06.010

## PERFORMING A CARDIAC CT IN A PATIENT WHO HAS VALVULAR DISEASE

### *Protocol Optimization*

As mentioned earlier, CAD assessment usually is the primary indication for cardiac CT in patients who have known VHD. Thus, imaging protocols usually are tailored to the evaluation of the coronary arteries. Before the contrast-enhanced CTA, a non-contrast CT often is acquired for the assessment of coronary calcium. These images also can be used to detect valvular calcification. Because of the lower radiation dose associated with prospective ECG gating, this approach usually is recommended for coronary calcium scoring.[6] Images typically are obtained at mid-diastole, when there is less coronary motion. This phase of the cardiac cycle also results in the lowest variability when quantifying aortic valvular calcium.[7] As reviewed later, determination of the degree of aortic valve calcification may provide important information with respect to valvular status and prognosis.

In contrast-enhanced coronary CTA, the use of the thinnest collimation available in the scanner is recommended for optimal visualization of the usually thin valve leaflets. Retrospective gating has been the most commonly used technique for ECG synchronization during coronary CTA. It also allows visualization of the heart in cine loops, which makes examination of biventricular function and valvular motion possible. Prospective ECG gating offers the distinct advantage of lower radiation exposure; however, it may be detrimental for the assessment of valvular pathology, because only valvular anatomy, but not motion, can be studied. Thus, if valvular evaluation is intended, retrospective ECG gating remains the technique of choice. Both the thinner collimation and retrospective gating capabilities are advantages of MDCT over electron beam CT, although the latter possesses superior temporal resolution and results in lower radiation exposure. When retrospective gating is used, implementation of ECG-based tube current modulation, commonly with maximal output during diastole and lower output during systole, leads to significant reductions in radiation dose.[8] This technique, however, also result can in suboptimal evaluation of stenotic lesions of the semilunar valves and of regurgitant lesions of the atrioventricular valves. Maximal output may be programmed to occur during systole if these abnormalities are suspected and if coronary evaluation is not hampered (ie, in patients who have faster heart rates). Alternatively, tube modulation may need to be avoided for optimal valvular evaluation.

In contrast administration, the standard use of a saline chaser bolus may limit visualization of right heart valves during coronary CTA. Therefore, optimized protocols that provide some degree of enhancement of the right cardiac chambers are preferred if these valves are to be studied. These methods include biphasic protocols that combine an infusion of contrast followed by a mixture of contrast and saline or contrast infusion at two different rates followed by saline and triphasic protocols that combine an infusion of contrast, followed by a mixture of contrast and saline, followed by saline.

### *Data Analysis*

With the aid of specialized computer software, the amount of calcium in the coronary arteries and in the cardiac valves can be quantified accurately. The Agatston score is the quantification method most commonly used in clinical practice, although the volume and mass methods have been proposed because of their superior reproducibility.[7] In ex vivo comparisons with the true calcium content of explanted valves, the amount of calcification is quantified precisely with electron beam CT.[9]

Valvular abnormalities also can be seen by playing a cine movie of multiphasic contrast-enhanced CTA reconstructions and analyzing the leaflet motion throughout the cardiac cycle. The leaflets of stenotic valves often are thickened, calcified, and display reduced opening (in diastole for atrioventricular valves and in systole for semilunar valves). Evaluation of regurgitant valves also may reveal structural abnormalities such as leaflet prolapse or incomplete coaptation. Stenosis severity usually is measured by finding the cardiac phase with the largest opening of the stenotic valve and using the method of valvular area planimetry. The inner contour of the valve opening is traced manually at the level of the leaflet tips and in a plane parallel to the annulus as determined from two orthogonal double-oblique views (**Fig. 1**). The same approach can be applied to the area of inadequate leaflet coaptation in regurgitant lesions, to quantify the regurgitant orifice. From the cine images, biventricular end-diastolic, end-systolic, and stroke volumes, ejection fractions, and myocardial mass also can be measured precisely.[10,11] These parameters are known to portend vital prognostic and therapeutic implications in patients who have VHD.[5] In isolated regurgitant lesions, the regurgitant volume also can be derived from the difference between the left and right ventricular stroke volumes.[12]

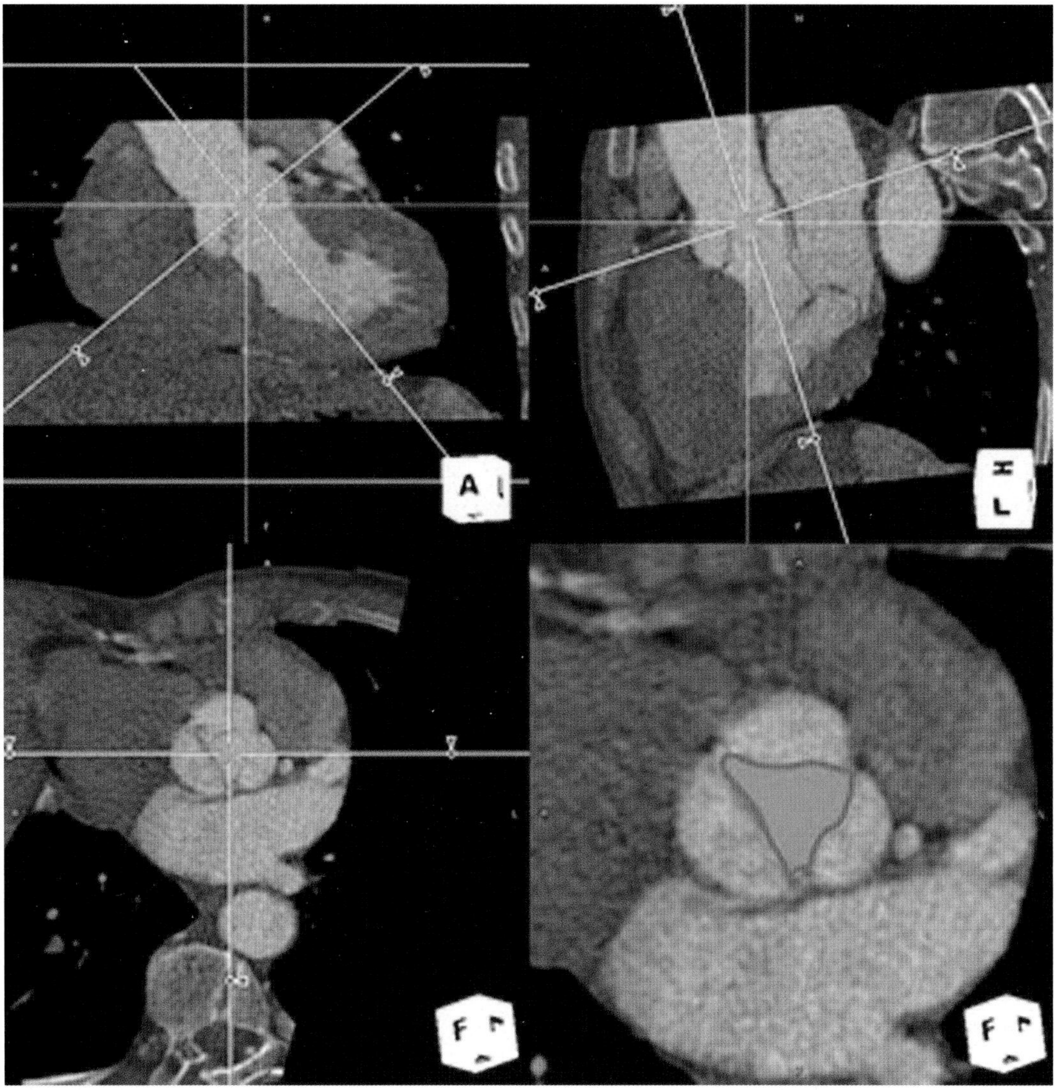

**Fig. 1.** Area planimetry of a tri-leaflet aortic valve during systole, in a cross-sectional view parallel to the annulus obtained from two orthogonal double-oblique views. The aortic valve area is shown in blue.

## INTERPRETING A CT STUDY IN PATIENTS WHO HAVE VALVULAR DISEASE

### *Cardiovascular Consequences of Valvular Disease*

Apart from the examination of the specific valves, there are secondary effects of VHD on the heart and the vascular system that can be evaluated with CT. Depending on the type and severity of valvular pathology, ventricular remodeling may occur. Stenoses of the semilunar valves lead to concentric hypertrophy with late-stage dilatation and post-stenotic enlargement of the ascending aorta or pulmonary artery. Regurgitation by any of the cardiac valves causes ventricular dilatation in the same side of the heart that also may be accompanied by eccentric hypertrophy. Stenotic and/or regurgitant lesions in the atrioventricular position usually create ipsilateral atrial dilatation. Pulmonary hypertension is a common consequence of VHD that typically leads to enlargement of the right heart chambers, pulmonary artery, and inferior and superior vena cava and to the development of ascites.[13] Pulmonary vein enlargement, pulmonary edema, and pleuro-pericardial effusions are all signs of increased pulmonary vein wedge pressures and left-sided heart failure.

### *Aortic Stenosis*

Aortic stenosis (AS) has several different pathologic mechanisms. The most common form in people under the age of 75 years is a congenitally bicuspid aortic valve, which occurs more commonly in men. A bicuspid aortic valve is the most prevalent cardiac congenital malformation and has a relatively high propensity for calcification and stenosis. Another important form of AS is senile degenerative calcification of the aortic valve, which is the leading cause of AS in persons over the age of 75 years and also is seen more frequently in men.[14] The risk factors for degenerative aortic valve disease are similar to those of atherosclerosis, including arterial hypertension, active smoking, and increased low-density lipoprotein and lipoprotein (a) cholesterol levels.[14] In the Multi-Ethnic Study of Atherosclerosis, 5723 subjects underwent CT scans for calcium scoring at baseline and at 2- or 3-year follow-ups. New incidence of aortic valve calcification was significantly increased in subjects who had metabolic syndrome.[15] The association of degenerative AS and CAD was highlighted in a study that evaluated 605 patients who had coronary calcium scores lower than 10. The presence of aortic valve calcium conveyed an increased risk (>10 fold) of ischemia detected by myocardial perfusion imaging.[16]

Calcification of the aortic valve is related directly to the development of AS. Moreover, the presence of moderate to severely calcified asymptomatic AS identifies a subgroup of patients more likely to develop symptoms or complications over the short term.[17] The amount of aortic valve calcification correlates directly with AS severity (**Table 1**). CT is an excellent modality for the evaluation of aortic valve calcification (**Fig. 2**). A valvular Agatston score of 1100 or higher has been associated with a 93% sensitivity and 82% specificity for the diagnosis of severe AS.[18] In addition, a score of 3700 or higher was found to have both a sensitivity and negative predictive value of 100%.[19] The location of the calcification seems to influence the severity of transvalvular gradients, and calcifications of the left noncoronary and the right–left commissures are most relevant.[20] Calcification in bicuspid aortic valves tends to occur at an earlier age, although there is no significant difference in the severity of calcification in bicuspid and tricuspid valves in patients who have symptomatic AS.[21]

With contrast-enhanced CT, it is possible to evaluate aortic valve morphology accurately, differentiating correctly between bicuspid and tricuspid aortic valves.[22] In addition, and as discussed earlier, the aortic valve area can be measured by planimetry. Planimetry is best performed 50 to 100 ms after the R peak, a phase that usually corresponds to the maximal valve opening and usually provides good imaging quality.[23] Aortic valve areas obtained from CT correlate strongly with transvalvular gradients or valve areas obtained with other modalities such as cardiac catheterization, echocardiography, or magnetic resonance (**Table 2**).

### *Aortic Regurgitation*

CT can be used similarly for the evaluation of aortic regurgitation (AR). The cause of AR often can be identified by evaluating the morphology, thickening, and calcification of the leaflets, their motion in cine loops, and the dimensions and characteristics of the aortic root. Potential mechanisms that can be detected with CT include insufficient leaflet coaptation in diastole (that is, visualization of the

**Table 1**
**Studies examining the relation between aortic valve calcification and aortic stenosis**

| Author, Reference | Number of Patients | CT Generation | Reference Standard | Method | Correlation (R Value) |
|---|---|---|---|---|---|
| Cowell et al.[19] | 157 | 2-slice | TTE | Peak gradient | 0.54 |
| Shavelle et al.[47] | 48 | EBCT | TTE | Peak velocities < and ≥ 2.5 m/s | AUC = 0.97 |
| Morgan-Hughes et al.[48] | 50 | 4-slice | TTE | Peak gradient<br>AVA (CE) | 0.77<br>0.73 |
| Messika-Zeitoun et al.[18] | 100 | EBCT | TTE | AVA (CE) | 0.79 |
| Koos et al.[49] | 72 | 16-slice | Catheterization | AVA (Gorlin)<br>PPG<br>Mean gradient | 0.67<br>0.70<br>0.72 |
| Koos et al.[2] | 21 | 4- and 16-slice | TTE | Peak gradient<br>Mean gradient | 0.47<br>0.45 |

*Abbreviations:* AUC, area under curve; AVA, aortic valve area; CE, continuity equation; EBCT, electron beam computed tomography; PPG, peak to peak gradient; TTE, transthoracic echocardiography.

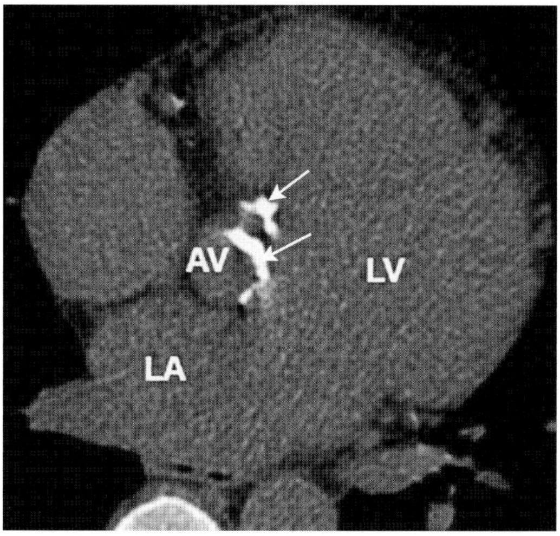


Fig. 2. Noncontrast CT acquired for coronary calcium scoring demonstrating aortic valve calcification (*arrows*). AV, aortic valve; LA, left atrium; LV, left ventricle.

regurgitant orifice) usually secondary to aortic root dilatation, leaflet prolapse, cusp perforation, or interposition of an intimal flap in cases of type A aortic dissection. When the regurgitant orifice is located centrally, it usually is secondary to dilatation of the aortic root. Regurgitant orifice areas measured by planimetry using MDCT (**Fig. 3**) correlate well with parameters of AR severity determined by echocardiography, such as the width of the vena contracta and the ratio of regurgitant jet to left ventricular outflow tract height.[24,25] In addition, in comparison with echocardiography, 64-slice MDCT has been shown to have high sensitivity (95%) and specificity (100%) for the detection of moderate and severe AR. Sensitivity decreases to 73%, but specificity remains high at 97% for the detection of mild AR when patients have severe aortic calcification or bicuspid aortic valves.[26]

## *Mitral Stenosis*

Worldwide, the most common cause of mitral stenosis continues to be rheumatic heart disease, although it is not seen as frequently in the United States. Diagnosis of rheumatic valve disease can be accomplished by visualization of the valvular apparatus and is characterized by retraction, thickening, and calcification of the mitral leaflets, chordae, and even papillary muscles. Cine imaging of the mitral valve using ECG-gated contrast-enhanced CT accurately visualizes valvular morphology.[27,28] Calcium scoring of the mitral valve annulus using CT is feasible also, although reproducibility is lower than that of the aortic valve.[29] The degree of calcification correlates with the severity of mitral valvular disease seen on echocardiography.[3] Mitral annular calcification also is associated with systemic atherosclerosis and has negative prognostic implications.[30] Contrast-enhanced CT is effective in evaluating mitral valve areas in patients who have mitral stenosis when compared with echocardiography. The area can be measured accurately by planimetry and has high reproducibility (**Fig. 4**).[31]

## *Mitral Regurgitation*

Mitral valve prolapse is a common cause of MR. It can be detected easily by contrast-enhanced CT when systolic frames or cine loops are reviewed. If mitral valve prolapse causes severe MR, visualization of which scallops of the leaflets prolapse into the left atrium can aid in the decision-making before surgery (**Fig. 5**). When MR is caused by prolapse, the direction of the regurgitant jet usually is eccentric, whereas mitral annulus dilatation leads to a central regurgitant orifice and flow jet caused by leaflet tenting and insufficient coaptation. The simultaneous evaluation of left ventricular contractility also may help elucidate whether segmental wall motion abnormalities in the insertion points of the papillary muscle contribute to valvular dysfunction in cases of ischemic MR. The severity of mitral insufficiency can be evaluated using MDCT by planimetry of the regurgitant orifice, which correlates significantly with transesophageal echocardiography (TEE).[32] Another approach for assessing MR severity is by obtaining the regurgitant volume. One technique validated with electron beam CT relies on quantifying the difference between the left ventricular stroke volume calculated from cine images and the forward stroke volume measured with the indicator dilution method.[33] Alternatively, the regurgitant volume can be obtained from the difference between left and right stroke volume derived from cine images. Quantification of regurgitant volumes or fractions is accurate only in isolated regurgitant lesions. In addition, knowledge of the presence of mitral annular or leaflet calcification can help the cardiothoracic surgeon determine the likelihood of successful repair or need for replacement before surgery.

## *Prosthetic Valves*

Visualization of mechanical prosthetic valves with echocardiography may be a challenge because of metal-related artifact. MDCT is capable of clearly depicting most mechanical cardiac valves, even without contrast administration, and of

**Table 2**
**Studies comparing aortic valve areas obtained from CT angiography and other imaging modalities**

| Study and Reference | Number of Patients | CT Generation | Reference Standard | Method | Correlation (R Value) | Bland Altman (Mean Bias – Limits of Agreement) ($cm^2$) |
|---|---|---|---|---|---|---|
| Feutchner et al.[50] | 30 | 16-slice | TTE | AVA (CE) | 0.89 | 0.04 (-0.20/0.29) |
| Alkadhi et al.[51] | 20 | 16-slice | TEE | AVA (CE) | 0.95 | 0.06 (-0.15/0.26) |
| | | | | AVA (planimetry) | 0.99 | — |
| | | | | Peak gradient | -0.74 | -0.08 (-0.32/0.16) |
| Bouvier et al.[52] | 30 | 16-slice | TTE (30p) | AVA (CE and/or Planimetry) | N/A | -0.07 (-0.4/0.25) |
| | | | TEE (3p) | — | — | — |
| Piers et al.[53] | 30 | EBCT | TTE | AVA (CE) | 0.60 | 0.51 (-0.4/1.42) |
| Feutchner et al.[54] | 36 | 64-slice | TTE (32p) | AVA (CE) | 0.88 | 0.06 (-0.35/0.40) |
| | | | — | Mean gradient | -0.68 | — |
| | | | — | Peak gradient | -0.67 | — |
| | | | TEE (10p) | AVA (planimetry) | 0.99 | -0.13 (-1.02/0.60) |
| Laissy et al.[55] | 40 | 16-slice | TTE | AVA (CE) | 0.77 | 0.05 (-0.26/0.36) |
| Tanaka et al.[56] | 29 | 16-slice | TTE | AVA (CE) | 0.96 | -0.03 (-0.21/0.15) |
| Pouleur et al.[22] | 27 | 40-slice | TEE (27p) | AVA (planimetry) | 0.98 | 0.10 (-0.5/0.7) |
| | | | TTE (27p) | AVA (CE) | 0.96 | 0.40 (-0.6/1.4) |
| | | | MRI (27p) | AVA (planimetry) | 0.98 | 0.00 (-0.6/0.6) |
| Lembcke et al.[57] | 32 | 40-slice | TTE (32p) | AVA (CE) | 0.86 | -0.30 (-0.82/0.22) |
| | | | CATH (32p) | AVA (Gorlin) | 0.90 | -0.24 (-0.68/0.20) |
| LaBounty et al.[58] | 80 | 64-slice | TEE (63 p) | AVA (planimetry) | 0.84 | -0.06 (-1.00/0.88) |
| | | | TTE (46 p) | AVA (CE) | 0.83 | 0.17 (-0.47/0.82) |

*Abbreviations:* AVA, aortic valve area; CATH, catheterization; CE, continuity equation; TEE, transesophageal echocardiography; TTE, transthoracic echocardiography.

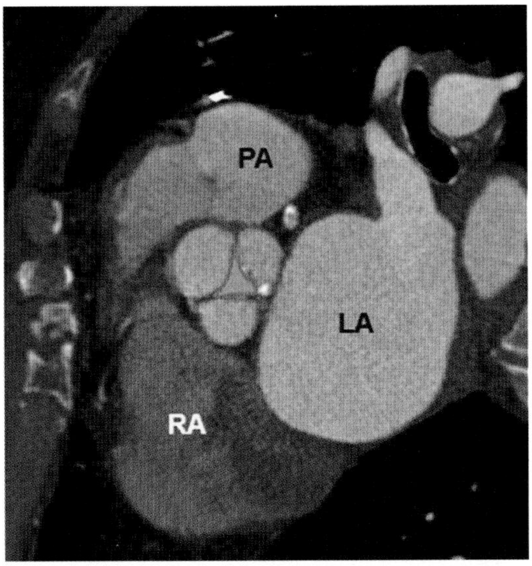


**Fig. 3.** Contrast-enhanced CT showing aortic valve in cross section during diastole. The regurgitant orifice area is demonstrated in blue. LA, left atrium; PA, pulmonary artery; RA, right atrium.

detecting abnormalities in the motion of the discs. Most mechanical valves used today are composed of two discs that open symmetrically when functioning properly (**Fig. 6**). In the evaluation of a single-disc prosthesis, the opening angle also can be calculated. Both types of valves have been evaluated by MDCT: valve function as well as opening and closing angles were compared with fluoroscopy and echocardiography. MDCT correlated significantly with both imaging modalities for two-disc mechanical valves; however, correlations for single-disc prostheses were significantly lower.[34] The role of CT in the assessment of bioprosthetic valves is similar to that of native VHD, potentially depicting abnormalities in leaflet motion and, importantly, degenerative calcification. Complications associated with prosthetic valves such as thrombosis or dehiscence also may be visualized with contrast-enhanced CT.

CT also can be of use in the assessment of valvular grafts. These grafts typically are implanted in the ascending aorta in patients who have aortic aneurysms and concomitant aortic valve disease. Besides allowing visualization of the valve prosthesis, CT provides accurate assessments of graft patency and size, as well as the presence of postsurgical complications.[35] Similarly, CT may have a role in patients who have aortic valve disease before or after undergoing a Ross procedure. This procedure consists of the replacement of a pathologic aortic valve with the patient's own healthy pulmonary trunk, which in turn is replaced by a cadaveric pulmonary homograft (**Fig. 7**). MDCT can be used pre- and postoperatively to evaluate the status of valves, great vessels, and grafts, including diameter, calcification, and functionality.

## *Infective Endocarditis*

Bacterial endocarditis is a life-threatening disease that can occur on native as well as prosthetic

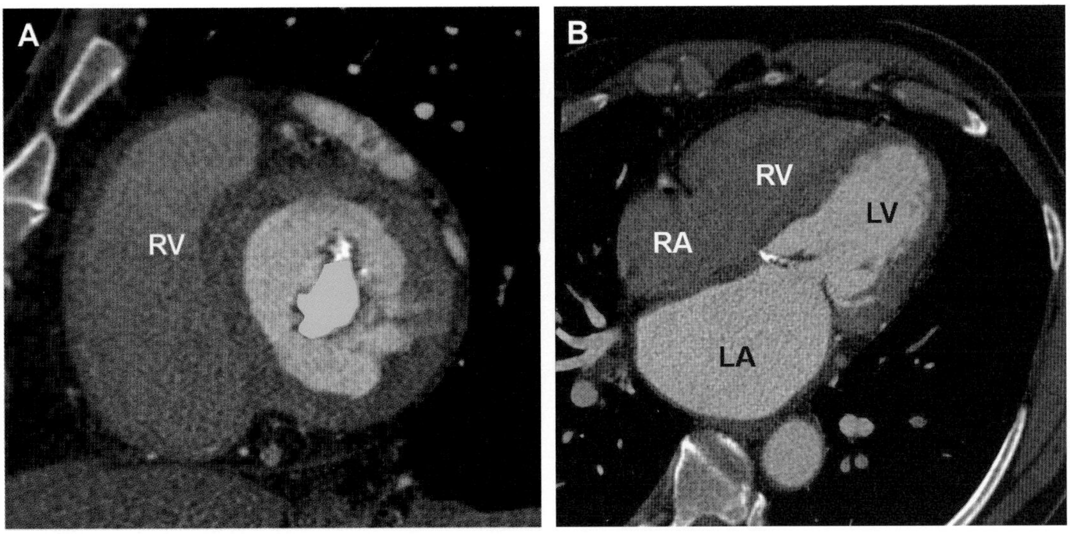


**Fig. 4.** (*A*) Contrast-enhanced short-axis view of the left ventricle and mitral valve during diastole. The image shows mild mitral stenosis as demonstrated by planimetry of the mitral valve area (*blue*). (*B*) Four-chamber view of the same stenotic mitral valve, where leaflet thickening and calcification can be noted. LA, left atrium; LV, left ventricle; RA, right atrium; RV, right ventricle.

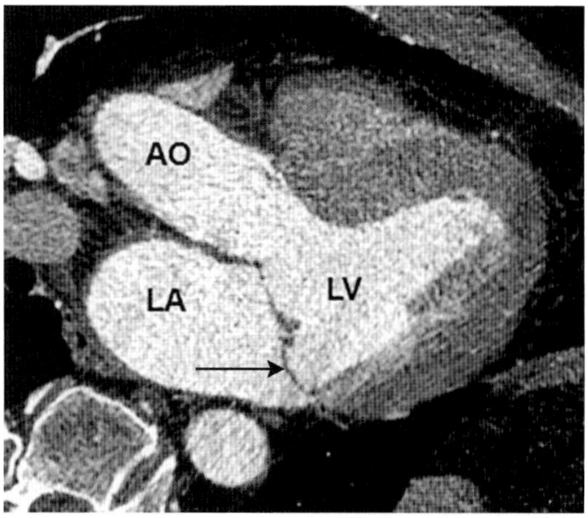


Fig. 5. End-systolic three-chamber view of a contrast-enhanced cardiac CT demonstrating prolapse of posterior mitral leaflet (*arrow*). AO, aorta; LA, left atrium; LV, left ventricle.

valves. It is associated with a mortality of up to 40%.[36] Diagnosis is achieved by direct visualization of valvular vegetations by TEE, which is the reference standard imaging modality. CT is inferior to echocardiography because of its lower temporal resolution. In many cases of infective endocarditis, however, perivalvular abscesses may be present also, and CT can be very useful for diagnosis (**Fig. 8**). Abscesses on CT appear as perivalvular fluid-filled collections, and by repeating the scan approximately 1 minute after contrast is given, retained contrast in the abscesses may be visualized.[37] A recent study compared MDCT with TEE and with intraoperative findings for the detection of infective endocarditis and abscesses. Thirty-seven patients suspected of having endocarditis were entered into the study. MDCT correctly identified 26 of 27 patients (96%) who had valvular vegetations and nine of nine patients (100%) who had abscesses. Compared with surgery findings, MDCT had a sensitivity of 96%, specificity of 97%, negative predictive value of 97%, and positive predictive value of 96% for the detection of vegetations or abscesses. The size of the vegetations as well as vegetation mobility correlated significantly between TEE and MDCT. Moreover, MDCT was superior to TEE in characterizing abscesses.[38]

## *Preoperative Coronary Artery Evaluation*

Another growing application of cardiac CT is preoperatively ruling out of significant CAD in patients undergoing valvular surgery. Coronary CTA is well established for the diagnosis of stable CAD in the outpatient setting with a 94% sensitivity and a 99% negative predictive in patients without known disease.[39] More recently, rapid rule-out protocols in the emergency department for acute chest pain also have demonstrated promising results.[40] Many hospital centers now are implementing CTA as a noninvasive alternative to CA for preoperative coronary evaluation of patients referred for valvular surgery, especially patients without known CAD and with low to intermediate pretest probability. Several studies have addressed this potential indication for CTA. One

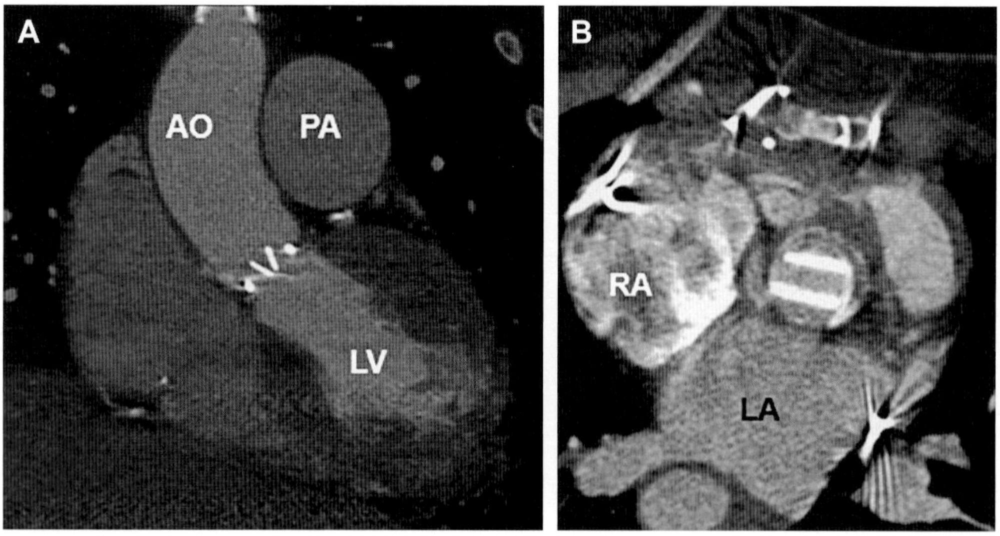


Fig. 6. (*A*) Coronal and (*B*) cross-sectional systolic views of a contrast-enhanced CT of the aorta demonstrating a mechanical valve in the aortic position with normal opening of both disks. AO, aorta; LA, left atrium; LV, left ventricle; PA, pulmonary artery; RA, right atrium.

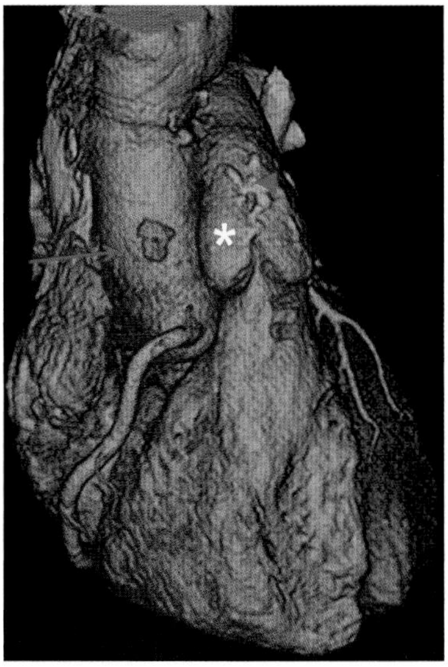


**Fig. 7.** Three-dimensional volume-rendered reconstruction of a contrast-enhanced CT of a patient who underwent a Ross surgical procedure. The pulmonary autograft is seen in the aortic position (*arrow*), and a homograft (*asterisk*) with degenerative calcification (*arrowhead*) is noted in the pulmonic position.

investigation examined the accuracy of 16-slice MDCT in 40 patients (mean age of 70 years) undergoing surgery for VHD of different etiologies. The patient-based sensitivity and specificity for the detection of significant coronary stenoses were 92% and 78%, respectively.[41] Another evaluation employed 64-slice MDCT in 50 patients (mean age of 54 years) undergoing valve replacement for AR. CTA demonstrated a sensitivity of 100%, specificity of 95%, and a negative predictive value of 100% when compared with CA. It was determined that preoperative CA could have been avoided in 70% of patients.[42] Two additional studies examined preoperative 16- and 64-slice coronary CTA in patients who had AS and mean ages of 68 and 70 years, respectively. The sensitivity and negative predictive value for the detection of significant stenosis were 100%; however, a moderate specificity and positive predictive value were found in both studies.[43,44] Further analysis demonstrated that excluding patients who had very high calcium scores (> 1000) improved specificity and positive predictive values significantly.[43,45] Finally, another study evaluated the safety of a strategy based on the results of coronary CTA in patients scheduled for valvular heart surgery. Individuals without significant lesions in the coronary arteries by MDCT were sent directly to valve surgery; those who had more than 50% stenotic plaques underwent CA. There were no cases of perioperative myocardial ischemia, infarction, or heart failure in the group of patients without significant CAD by MDCT.[46]

These studies show that coronary CTA may be used safely to rule out significant CAD and avoid unneeded invasive procedures. Nonetheless, individuals who have VHD often have relative contraindications for MDCT (eg, arrhythmia), which may preclude the examination in a significant proportion of cases.[41,44] Also, the use of coronary CTA in patients who have AS merits special

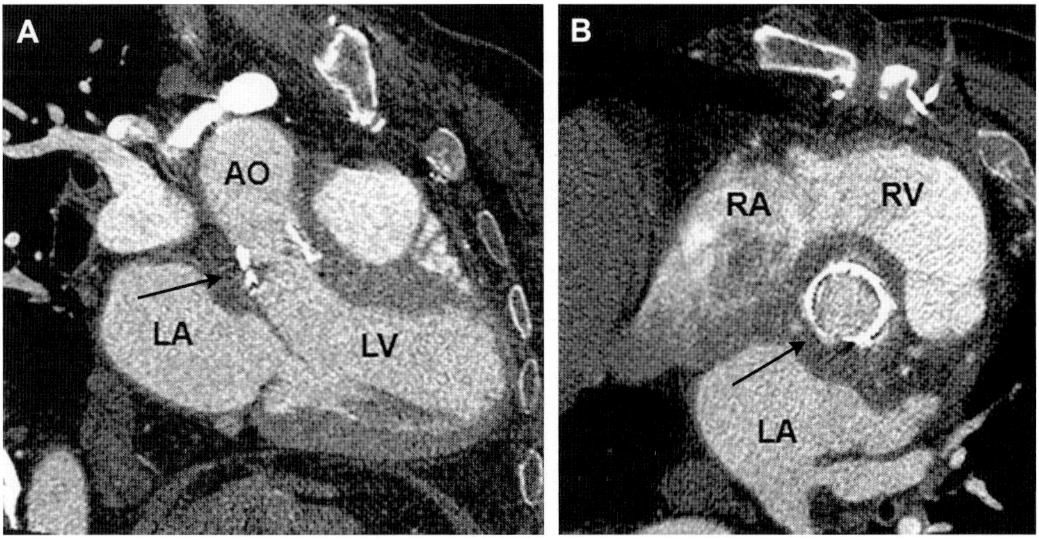


**Fig. 8.** (*A*) Three-chamber view of a contrast-enhanced cardiac CT demonstrating a bioprosthetic valve in the aortic position. The arrow marks a perivalvular abscess. (*B*) Same abscess visualized in a cross-sectional view (*arrow*). AO, aorta; LA, left atrium; LV, left ventricle; RA, right atrium; RV, right ventricle.

consideration. As mentioned earlier, patients who have AS tend to be elderly and commonly have extensive CAD and coronary calcification. Indeed, more than one third of the patients who undergo aortic valve replacement for AS have concurrent significant CAD.[5] As a result, the diagnostic yield of coronary CTA may be lower in these patients.[43–45] In addition, administration of intravenous beta-blockade may be hazardous in the context of severe AS. Although beta-blockers have not been associated with complication in recent studies,[43,44] cautious administration seems prudent. Thus, preoperative coronary CTA may be particularly useful in individuals who have either mitral disease or AR.

## SUMMARY

CT is an accurate and reasonable alternative modality for valvular imaging when echocardiography is unable to provide a complete characterization of VHD and magnetic resonance is unavailable or contraindicated. Even if coronary evaluation is the primary indication, important information regarding valvular anatomy and function can be derived from CT. Calcification is a common CT finding in various valvular abnormalities and carries important diagnostic and prognostic value. In addition to calcification, valvular morphology, stenosis, and regurgitation are evaluable on contrast-enhanced scans, with good correlation with echocardiography and other techniques. If valvular assessment is intended, however, adaptation of the protocol for optimal visualization of the valves is recommended. In addition, preoperative coronary CTA for patients scheduled for cardiac valve surgery seems to be reliable and has the potential to eliminate the need for cardiac catheterization in a substantial proportion of patients.

## REFERENCES

1. Lippert JA, White CS, Mason AC, et al. Calcification of aortic valve detected incidentally on CT scans: prevalence and clinical significance. AJR Am J Roentgenol 1995;164:73–7.
2. Koos R, Kuhl HP, Muhlenbruch G, et al. Prevalence and clinical importance of aortic valve calcification detected incidentally on CT scans: comparison with echocardiography. Radiology 2006;241:76–82.
3. Mahnken AH, Muhlenbruch G, Das M, et al. MDCT detection of mitral valve calcification: prevalence and clinical relevance compared with echocardiography. AJR Am J Roentgenol 2007;188:1264–9.
4. Nkomo VT, Gardin JM, Skelton TN, et al. Burden of valvular heart diseases: a population-based study. Lancet 2006;368:1005–11.
5. Bonow RO, Carabello BA, Chatterjee K, et al. 2008 Focused update incorporated into the ACC/AHA 2006 guidelines for the management of patients with valvular heart disease: a report of the American College of Cardiology/American Heart Association Task Force on Practice Guidelines (Writing Committee to Revise the 1998 Guidelines for the Management of Patients With Valvular Heart Disease): endorsed by the Society of Cardiovascular Anesthesiologists, Society for Cardiovascular Angiography and Interventions, and Society of Thoracic Surgeons. Circulation 2008;118:e523–661.
6. McCollough CH, Ulzheimer S, Halliburton SS, et al. Coronary artery calcium: a multi-institutional, multimanufacturer international standard for quantification at cardiac CT. Radiology 2007;243:527–38.
7. Ruhl KM, Das M, Koos R, et al. Variability of aortic valve calcification measurement with multislice spiral computed tomography. Invest Radiol 2006;41:370–3.
8. Jakobs TF, Becker CR, Ohnesorge B, et al. Multislice helical CT of the heart with retrospective ECG gating: reduction of radiation exposure by ECG-controlled tube current modulation. Eur Radiol 2002;12:1081–6.
9. Pohle K, Dimmler A, Feyerer R, et al. Quantification of aortic valve calcification with electron beam tomography: a histomorphometric validation study. Invest Radiol 2004;39:230–4.
10. Orakzai SH, Orakzai RH, Nasir K, et al. Assessment of cardiac function using multidetector row computed tomography. J Comput Assist Tomogr 2006;30:555–63.
11. Plumhans C, Muhlenbruch G, Rapaee A, et al. Assessment of global right ventricular function on 64-MDCT compared with MRI. AJR Am J Roentgenol 2008;190:1358–61.
12. Reiter SJ, Rumberger JA, Stanford W, et al. Quantitative determination of aortic regurgitant volumes in dogs by ultrafast computed tomography. Circulation 1987;76:728–35.
13. Boxt LM. CT of valvular heart disease. Int J Cardiovasc Imaging 2005;21:105–13.
14. Stewart BF, Siscovick D, Lind BK, et al. Clinical factors associated with calcific aortic valve disease. Cardiovascular Health Study. J Am Coll Cardiol 1997;29:630–4.
15. Katz R, Budoff MJ, Takasu J, et al. Relationship of metabolic syndrome with incident aortic valve calcium and aortic valve calcium progression: the multi-ethnic study of atherosclerosis. Diabetes 2009;58:813–9.
16. Ho J, FitzGerald S, Cannaday J, et al. Relation of aortic valve calcium to myocardial ischemic perfusion in individuals with a low coronary artery calcium score. Am J Cardiol 2007;99:1535–7.

17. Rosenhek R, Binder T, Porenta G, et al. Predictors of outcome in severe, asymptomatic aortic stenosis. N Engl J Med 2000;343:611–7.
18. Messika-Zeitoun D, Aubry MC, Detaint D, et al. Evaluation and clinical implications of aortic valve calcification measured by electron-beam computed tomography. Circulation 2004;110:356–62.
19. Cowell SJ, Newby DE, Burton J, et al. Aortic valve calcification on computed tomography predicts the severity of aortic stenosis. Clin Radiol 2003;58:712–6.
20. Liu F, Coursey CA, Grahame-Clarke C, et al. Aortic valve calcification as an incidental finding at CT of the elderly: severity and location as predictors of aortic stenosis. AJR Am J Roentgenol 2006;186:342–9.
21. Ferda J, Linhartova K, Kreuzberg B. Comparison of the aortic valve calcium content in the bicuspid and tricuspid stenotic aortic valve using nonenhanced 64-detector-row-computed tomography with prospective ECG-triggering. Eur J Radiol 2008;68:471–5.
22. Pouleur AC, le Polain de Waroux JB, Pasquet A, et al. Aortic valve area assessment: multidetector CT compared with cine MR imaging and transthoracic and transesophageal echocardiography. Radiology 2007;244:745–54.
23. Abbara S, Pena AJ, Maurovich-Horvat P, et al. Feasibility and optimization of aortic valve planimetry with MDCT. AJR Am J Roentgenol 2007;188:356–60.
24. Alkadhi H, Desbiolles L, Husmann L, et al. Aortic regurgitation: assessment with 64-section CT. Radiology 2007;245:111–21.
25. Jassal DS, Shapiro MD, Neilan TG, et al. 64-slice multidetector computed tomography (MDCT) for detection of aortic regurgitation and quantification of severity. Invest Radiol 2007;42:507–12.
26. Feuchtner GM, Dichtl W, Muller S, et al. 64-MDCT for diagnosis of aortic regurgitation in patients referred to CT coronary angiography. AJR Am J Roentgenol 2008;191:W1–7.
27. Alkadhi H, Bettex D, Wildermuth S, et al. Dynamic cine imaging of the mitral valve with 16-MDCT: a feasibility study. AJR Am J Roentgenol 2005;185:636–46.
28. Willmann JK, Kobza R, Roos JE, et al. ECG-gated multi-detector row CT for assessment of mitral valve disease: initial experience. Eur Radiol 2002;12: 2662–9.
29. Budoff MJ, Takasu J, Katz R, et al. Reproducibility of CT measurements of aortic valve calcification, mitral annulus calcification, and aortic wall calcification in the multi-ethnic study of atherosclerosis. Acad Radiol 2006;13:166–72.
30. Allison MA, Cheung P, Criqui MH, et al. Mitral and aortic annular calcification are highly associated with systemic calcified atherosclerosis. Circulation 2006;113:861–6.
31. Messika-Zeitoun D, Serfaty JM, Laissy JP, et al. Assessment of the mitral valve area in patients with mitral stenosis by multislice computed tomography. J Am Coll Cardiol 2006;48:411–3.
32. Alkadhi H, Wildermuth S, Bettex DA, et al. Mitral regurgitation: quantification with 16-detector row CT–initial experience. Radiology 2006;238:454–63.
33. Lembcke A, Borges AC, Dushe S, et al. Assessment of mitral valve regurgitation at electron-beam CT: comparison with Doppler echocardiography. Radiology 2005;236:47–55.
34. Konen E, Goitein O, Feinberg MS, et al. The role of ECG-gated MDCT in the evaluation of aortic and mitral mechanical valves: initial experience. AJR Am J Roentgenol 2008;191:26–31.
35. Sundaram B, Quint LE, Patel S, et al. CT appearance of thoracic aortic graft complications. AJR Am J Roentgenol 2007;188:1273–7.
36. Bashore TM, Cabell C, Fowler V Jr. Update on infective endocarditis. Curr Probl Cardiol 2006;31: 274–352.
37. Gilkeson RC, Markowitz AH, Balgude A, et al. MDCT evaluation of aortic valvular disease. AJR Am J Roentgenol 2006;186:350–60.
38. Feuchtner GM, Stolzmann P, Dichtl W, et al. Multislice computed tomography in infective endocarditis: comparison with transesophageal echocardiography and intraoperative findings. J Am Coll Cardiol 2009; 53:436–44.
39. Budoff MJ, Dowe D, Jollis JG, et al. Diagnostic performance of 64-multidetector row coronary computed tomographic angiography for evaluation of coronary artery stenosis in individuals without known coronary artery disease: results from the prospective multicenter ACCURACY (Assessment by Coronary Computed Tomographic Angiography of Individuals Undergoing Invasive Coronary Angiography) trial. J Am Coll Cardiol 2008;52:1724–32.
40. Goldstein JA, Gallagher MJ, O'Neill WW, et al. A randomized controlled trial of multi-slice coronary computed tomography for evaluation of acute chest pain. J Am Coll Cardiol 2007;49:863–71.
41. Reant P, Brunot S, Lafitte S, et al. Predictive value of noninvasive coronary angiography with multidetector computed tomography to detect significant coronary stenosis before valve surgery. Am J Cardiol 2006;97:1506–10.
42. Scheffel H, Leschka S, Plass A, et al. Accuracy of 64-slice computed tomography for the preoperative detection of coronary artery disease in patients with chronic aortic regurgitation. Am J Cardiol 2007;100: 701–6.
43. Gilard M, Cornily JC, Pennec PY, et al. Accuracy of multislice computed tomography in the preoperative assessment of coronary disease in patients with aortic valve stenosis. J Am Coll Cardiol 2006;47:2020–4.
44. Meijboom WB, Mollet NR, Van Mieghem CA, et al. Pre-operative computed tomography coronary angiography to detect significant coronary artery

disease in patients referred for cardiac valve surgery. J Am Coll Cardiol 2006;48:1658–65.
45. Manghat NE, Morgan-Hughes GJ, Broadley AJ, et al. 16-detector row computed tomographic coronary angiography in patients undergoing evaluation for aortic valve replacement: comparison with catheter angiography. Clin Radiol 2006;61:749–57.
46. Russo V, Gostoli V, Lovato L, et al. Clinical value of multidetector CT coronary angiography as a preoperative screening test before non-coronary cardiac surgery. Heart 2007;93:1591–8.
47. Shavelle DM, Budoff MJ, Buljubasic N, et al. Usefulness of aortic valve calcium scores by electron beam computed tomography as a marker for aortic stenosis. Am J Cardiol 2003;92:349–53.
48. Morgan-Hughes GJ, Owens PE, Roobottom CA, et al. Three dimensional volume quantification of aortic valve calcification using multislice computed tomography. Heart 2003;89:1191–4.
49. Koos R, Mahnken AH, Sinha AM, et al. Aortic valve calcification as a marker for aortic stenosis severity: assessment on 16-MDCT. AJR Am J Roentgenol 2004;183:1813–8.
50. Feuchtner GM, Dichtl W, Friedrich GJ, et al. Multislice computed tomography for detection of patients with aortic valve stenosis and quantification of severity. J Am Coll Cardiol 2006;47:1410–7.
51. Alkadhi H, Wildermuth S, Plass A, et al. Aortic stenosis: comparative evaluation of 16-detector row CT and echocardiography. Radiology 2006;240:47–55.
52. Bouvier E, Logeart D, Sablayrolles JL, et al. Diagnosis of aortic valvular stenosis by multislice cardiac computed tomography. Eur Heart J 2006;27:3033–8.
53. Piers LH, Dikkers R, Tio RA, et al. A comparison of echocardiographic and electron beam computed tomographic assessment of aortic valve area in patients with valvular aortic stenosis. Int J Cardiovasc Imaging 2007;23:781–8.
54. Feuchtner GM, Muller S, Bonatti J, et al. Sixty-four slice CT evaluation of aortic stenosis using planimetry of the aortic valve area. AJR Am J Roentgenol 2007;189:197–203.
55. Laissy JP, Messika-Zeitoun D, Serfaty JM, et al. Comprehensive evaluation of preoperative patients with aortic valve stenosis: usefulness of cardiac multidetector computed tomography. Heart 2007;93:1121–5.
56. Tanaka H, Shimada K, Yoshida K, et al. The simultaneous assessment of aortic valve area and coronary artery stenosis using 16-slice multidetector-row computed tomography in patients with aortic stenosis comparison with echocardiography. Circ J 2007;71:1593–8.
57. Lembcke A, Thiele H, Lachnitt A, et al. Precision of forty slice spiral computed tomography for quantifying aortic valve stenosis: comparison with echocardiography and validation against cardiac catheterization. Invest Radiol 2008;43:719–28.
58. LaBounty TM, Sundaram B, Agarwal P, et al. Aortic valve area on 64-MDCT correlates with transesophageal echocardiography in aortic stenosis. AJR Am J Roentgenol 2008;191:1652–8.

# Left Ventricular Function, Myocardial Perfusion and Viability

Yasuyuki Kobayashi, MD[a,c], Albert C. Lardo, PhD[a,b], Yasuo Nakajima, MD, PhD[c], Joao A.C. Lima, MD[a,d], Richard T. George, MD[a,*]

**KEYWORDS**

• Cardiac computed tomography • Function
• Perfusion • Viability • Myocardial infarction

Visualization of the coronary arteries using diastolic reconstruction with helical scanning CT was first reported in 1995[1] and the first report of ECG-gated multidetector row CT (MDCT) for the noninvasive detection of coronary artery stenosis and cardiac structure was published in 2000.[2] Over the past decade, improvements in temporal and spatial resolution, along with wider detector coverage, have expanded the use of MDCT to the assessment of cardiac function, perfusion, and viability, in addition to noninvasive coronary angiography. Cardiac CT is now poised to revolutionize the practice of cardiology. The comprehensive assessment of left ventricular (LV) function and myocardial perfusion, as well as coronary CT angiography, has previously been reported.[3,4] Further technologic developments, such as wide-area CT (ie, 256-slice and 320-row detector CT), dual-source, flat-panel detector CT, and hybrids of these technologies promise to improve the capabilities of cardiac CT in the assessment of cardiac function, perfusion, and viability.[5–9]

## FUNCTIONAL ANALYSIS

Accurate, noninvasive assessment of ventricular function is fundamental to provide excellent care to patients with cardiovascular diseases. Global and regional LV function can be assessed using different invasive modalities, such as cine-ventriculography, and noninvasive modalities, such as echocardiography, cine MRI, ECG-gated single-photon emission computed tomography (SPECT), and positron emission tomography (PET) in clinical practice.

Cardiac MDCT imaging using retrospective ECG-gating acquires data throughout the cardiac cycle from systole to diastole, which allows images to be reconstructed at multiple cardiac phases of the R-R interval. Image data are usually reconstructed from 0% to 90% of the cardiac cycle at 10% intervals for the assessment of cardiac function (**Fig. 1**A). Endocardial and epicardial borders can be outlined using either manual or automated contour-detection algorithms.[10] By using these contours, myocardial mass, end-systolic volume (ESV) and end-diastolic volume (EDV), stroke volume, cardiac output, and ejection fraction (EF) can be calculated (**Fig. 1**B).

MRI is the current gold standard for assessing LV function. Studies comparing MDCT and MRI show measurements of stroke volume, ESV and EDV, EF, and regional wall motion scores are strongly correlated.[10–15] Many small comparative

[a] Department of Medicine, Division of Cardiology, The Johns Hopkins University School of Medicine, 600 North Wolfe Street, Blalock 524 Baltimore, MD 21287, USA
[b] Department of Biomedical Engineering, The Johns Hopkins University School of Medicine, 600 North Wolfe Street, Blalock 524 Baltimore, MD 21287, USA
[c] Department of Radiology, St. Marianna University School of Medicine, 2-16-1 Sugao, Miyamae-ku, Kawasaki, Kanagawa, 216-8511, Japan
[d] Department of Radiology, The Johns Hopkins University School of Medicine, 600 North Wolfe Street, Blalock 524 Baltimore, MD 21287, USA
* Corresponding author.
*E-mail address:* rgeorge3@jhmi.edu (R.T. George).

Cardiol Clin 27 (2009) 645–654
doi:10.1016/j.ccl.2009.06.004

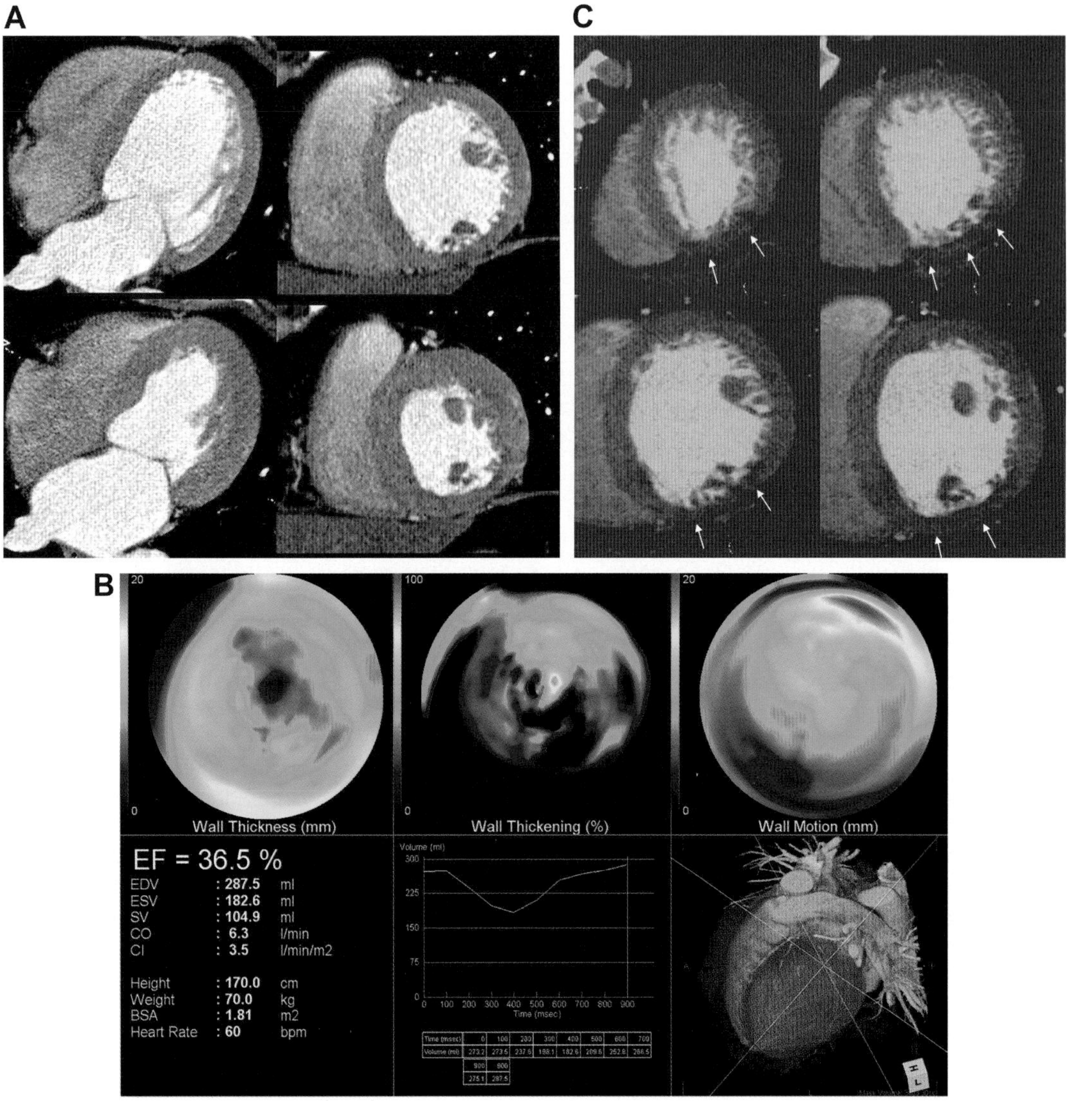


**Fig. 1.** Chronic myocardial infarction of the inferior wall. (*A*) Reconstruction of the endo-diastolic and endo-systolic phases. Akinesis and thinning of the inferior and inferolateral wall is noted. (*B*) Functional assessment using MDCT revealed a moderately reduced global ejection fraction of the left ventricle (EF: 37%). Bull's eye images show decreased wall thickening and wall motion of inferior wall. (*C*) Adenosine stress-perfusion CT images shows hypo-enhanced area in inferoseptal, inferior, and inferolateral wall, corresponding to prior myocardial infarction (*arrows*).

studies suggest that CT has good agreement with MRI and that it could potentially be an alternative to MRI in some patients, especially those with implantable cardiac devices. Furthermore, inter-observer variation of global LV function was reported to be 2% to 8.5% for LV-EDV, 4 to 10.8% for LV-ESV, and 2% to 9.6% for EF, within the range of other modalities.[13,16,17] However, MDCT does have a tendency to overestimate volumetric measurements.[10–17] In addition to LV function, MDCT is also well suited to measure right ventricular mass and function,[18,19] and left atrial measurements.[19] However, because of limits in temporal resolution, MDCT is inferior in the measurement of dynamic functional parameters, such as peak filling rate, peak ejection rate, time to peak ejection rate, and time from end-systole to peak filling rate when compared with MRI.

The use of CT to assess ventricular function is limited by the use of contrast and radiation, and temporal resolution. By using a phantom, Mahnken and colleagues[20,21] reported that enhanced temporal resolution improves the quantification of LV volumetric parameters, and dual-source CT allows more reliable quantification of ventricular function than single-source CT. Currently, quantitative assessments using dual-source CT have reported that dual-source CT has a strong correlation with MRI regarding cardiac-function analysis.[22–24] Brodoefel and colleagues[22] reported good correlation for peak ejection rate and peak filling rate. In the near future, its widespread availability and improved temporal resolution suggest that MDCT will have expansive use in clinical setting.

## MYOCARDIAL PERFUSION IMAGING

Perfusion imaging adds valuable prgnostic value beyond the invasive coronary angiogram and the identification and quantification of ischemia can risk-stratify patients for medical versus invasive therapies.[25] Hybrid imaging systems combining MDCT with SPECT or PET have been developed, but require the cost associated with hybridizing two imaging modalities and added ionizing radiation.[26,27] On the other hand, MDCT alone has the potential to not only detect a morphologic stenosis of the coronary artery, but also its functional significance.

Previously, investigators showed that electron-beam CT could accurately measure myocardial blood flow. Using serial images of the left ventricle, myocardial blood flow can be accurately quantified by applying various adaptations of indicator-dilution theory.[28–31]

Likewise, the current generation of MDCT scanning systems can be programmed to acquire the sequential datasets in dynamic mode and track the kinetics of iodinated contrast in the myocardium and LV blood pool. For the quantification of myocardial blood flow, sequential ECG-gated images are acquired without table movement during at least every second heart beat. Using dynamic time-attenuation curves, robust metrics of myocardial blood flow can be derived using up-slope and model-based deconvolution methods, with excellent correlations with the gold standard for myocardial blood flow, microspheres ($R^2$ = 0.91, $P<.0001$) (**Fig. 2**).[32] In addition, quantitative parameters of microvascular function can be derived from dynamic MDCT imaging.[33]

Dynamic MDCT perfusion imaging, however, has several limitations using today's 64-slice MDCT scanners. The current generation of 64-slice MDCT scanners has limited coverage in the *z*-axis, with coverage limited to 28 mm to 40 mm depending on scanner manufacturer. In addition, serial imaging of the heart requiring multiple X-ray exposures over time require high radiation dose, making the application of dynamic MDCT for myocardial perfusion difficult. The recent introduction of dynamic-volume 320-row detector CT has made whole-heart dynamic imaging possible. However, it is currently unknown whether prospective ECG-gated protocols with tube-current modulation will be capable of significant radiation dose reductions to make dynamic myocardial perfusion imaging feasible.

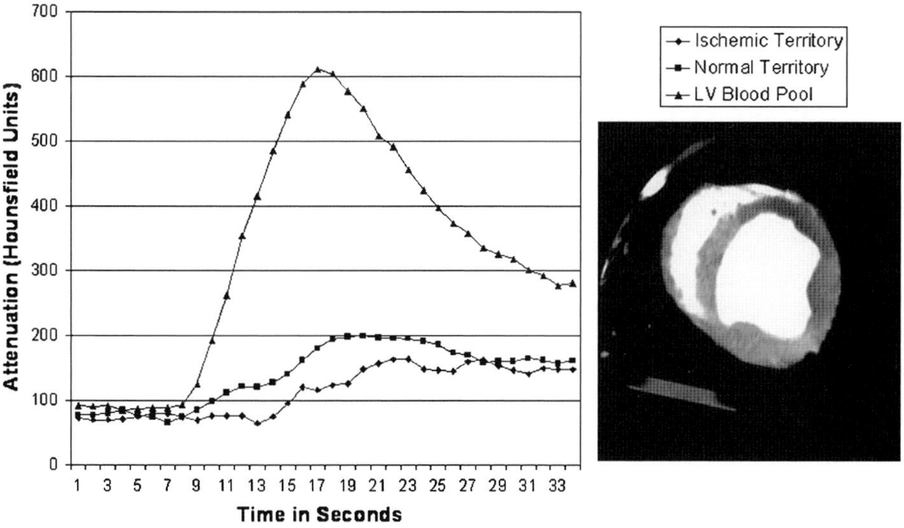


**Fig. 2.** Myocardial enhancement after the administration of contrast medium in a canine model of left anterior descending artery (LAD) stenosis. The time-attenuation curve for the LV blood pool, and the normal and ischemic territories obtained during adenosine stress are shown on the right. CT myocardial perfusion imaging at peak contrast enhancement is shown on the right. Note the hypo-enhanced region in the anterior wall.

A feasible alternative to dynamic MDCT perfusion imaging is performing CT perfusion imaging using helical MDCT protocols. Recently, several articles have been published demonstrating that ischemic myocardium can be detected by pharmacologic-stress MDCT perfusion performed with helical mode scanning (**Fig. 3**).[34–38] Recent studies from the authors' institution have shown in a canine model of LAD stenosis that MDCT angiography, performed during adenosine infusion with the scanner programmed in helical mode, can detect differences in myocardial perfusion.[36–38] In addition, studies from the authors' institution have established the feasibility of CT perfusion imaging using wide-area detector CT using 256- and 320-row detector CT.[37,39,40]

In a study that implemented both 64-detector helical CT and 256-row detector CT in 43 patients with suspicion of coronary artery disease based on abnormal radionuclide myocardial perfusion imaging, the authors were able to show that transmural differences in myocardial perfusion had a moderate inverse relationship with percent-diameter stenosis calculated with quantitative coronary angiography ($R = -0.63$, $P<.001$). In addition, the combination of CT angiography and adenosine stress-CT perfusion imaging demonstrated excellent accuracy in detecting obstructive atherosclerosis causing myocardial perfusion abnormalities, when compared with the combined gold standard of invasive angiography and radionuclide perfusion imaging with a sensitivity, specificity, positive-, and negative-predictive value of 86%, 92%, 92%, and 85%, respectively. Studies of rest and stress-CT perfusion imaging using 320-row CT are ongoing at the authors' institution.[39]

## MYOCARDIAL INFARCTION AND VIABILITY IMAGING

Visualization of myocardial infarction and viability is a very important concept, because dysfunctional—but viable—myocardium has the potential for functional recovery after revascularization. Noninvasive methods to assess myocardial viability is of very great importance and allows the selection of patients who will benefit from invasive coronary revascularization, such as percutaneous coronary angioplasty or coronary artery bypass grafting.[38,39] Several methods to assess myocardial viability, such as SPECT, PET and MRI, have been established.[41–44] MRI has evolved as a clinically accepted gold standard to assess myocardial viability, which has the advantage of better spatial resolution and the capability of differentiating transmural to subendocardial infarction, in contrast to SPECT and PET.

MDCT with iodinated intravenous contrast, similar to MRI, is useful for myocardial viability imaging. The pharmacokinetic behavior of gadolinium chelates is somewhat similar to that of iodinated contrast agents. Iodinated intravenous contrast agents primarily remain intravascular during the early part of first-pass circulation and then later diffuse into the extravascular space.[45–47] By MDCT measurement using iodinated contrast agents, myocardial attenuation has a direct linear

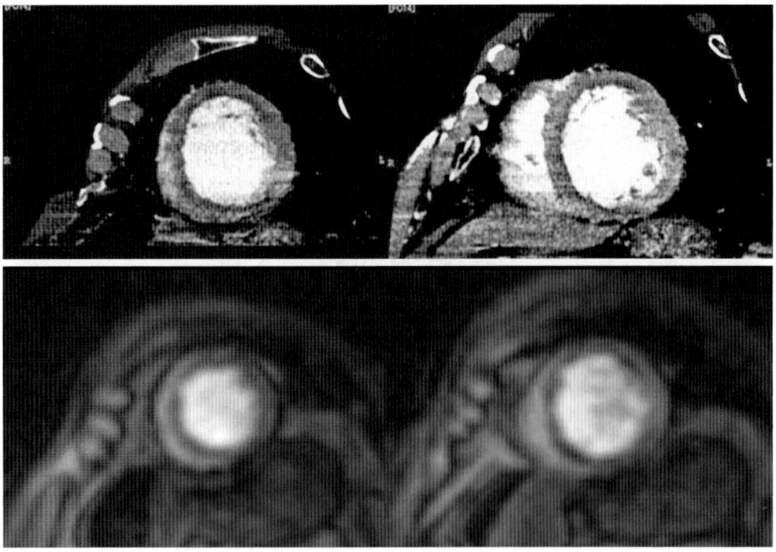

Fig. 3. Pharmacologic stress perfusion with MDCT (*top*) and MRI (*bottom*) in a patient with angina pectoris. The area of early defect in stress-perfusion MDCT correctly corresponds to the area in stress-perfusion MRI.

relationship to tissue iodine concentration.[32] The improved spatial resolution by MDCT reduces the partial volume artifacts and, therefore, has the potential for more accurate volumetric sizing of myocardial infarcts, as compared with other imaging modalities, such as such as SPECT, PET, and MRI.[48]

## First-pass Perfusion MDCT

These characteristics provide an opportunity to detect hypo-enhanced areas, early after contrast injection, which signify hypo-perfusion, and conversely detect hyper-enhanced areas, later after contrast injection, which signify damaged myocardium, such as acute myocardial infarction or myocardial scar.

During first-pass circulation of intravenous contrast medium, myocardial infarction can be detected as the presence of an early defect characterized as an area of hypo-enhanced myocardium (see **Figs. 1** and **4**). Nikolaou and colleagues[49] were the first to demonstrate in a systematic method the significance of early defects in patients. MDCT accurately detected the presence of myocardial infarction in 90% of cases, compared with biplane ventriculography. In addition, a recent study using a porcine model of LAD occlusion showed that MDCT could be used to detect acute myocardial infarction.[50] This study showed that the size of an early perfusion defect correlated well with the extent of myocardial infarction shown by postmortem triphenyltetrazolium chloride (TTC) staining. More recently, 16-detector CT was compared with delayed-enhanced MRI for the detection of chronic infarcts. In a group of 30 patients that underwent MDCT angiography, first-pass MDCT detected 10 out of 11 infarcts noted on delayed-enhanced MRI, yielding a sensitivity, specificity, and accuracy of 91%, 79%, and 83%, respectively.[51]

Nieman and colleagues[52] reported that early hypo-enhanced areas were recognized on all MDCT compared with MRI, and hypo-enhanced areas at first-pass MDCT correlated well with those at first-pass MRI, but the detection of a subtle subendocardial infarction might be difficult by MDCT because of the weaker contrast between the normal and infarcted myocardium when compared with MRI. Choe and colleagues[53] showed in a study of 63 patients that MDCT revealed prior myocardial infarction during

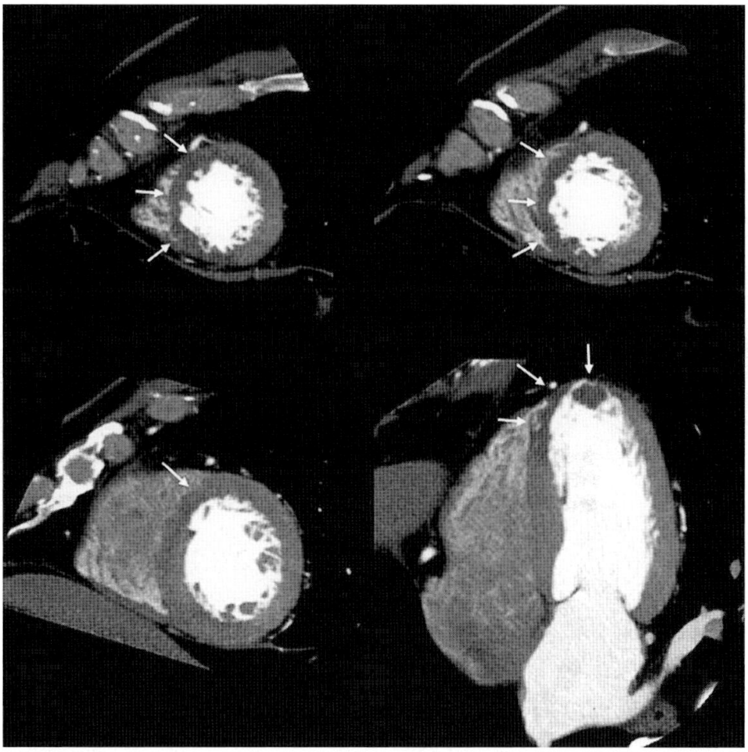

**Fig. 4.** Chronic myocardial infarction of distal septal, distal anterior, and apical walls. Note the hypo-enhanced areas within these walls (*arrows*). Thinning of the distal septum and apical walls with a thrombus noted in the apex.

first-phase contrast enhacement in all cases except for one (1.3%). There was no significant difference in the average lesion volume between perfusion MRI and early CT.

Wada and colleagues[54] reported that first-pass MDCT could be useful for the assessment of viability. In this study, the transmural infarction group by first-pass perfusion MDCT showed poor recovery of anterior wall motion at 6 months after onset of acute myocardial infarction, whereas the subendocardial infarction group exhibited good recovery of regional and global LV function.

## *Delayed-enhanced MDCT*

Delayed-enhanced MRI is well validated in the detection of myocardial viability.[42,55] Similar to gadolinium, iodinated contrast medium is preferentially taken up by irreversibly damaged myocytes and fibrotic myocardial scar over time. The pharmacokinetic behavior of gadolinium chelates is somewhat similar to that of iodinated contrast agents, so delayed-enhanced MDCT is also useful for myocardial viability imaging.

In a canine model of LAD occlusion and reperfusion after 90 minutes, Lardo and colleagues[56] demonstrated that the spatial extent of cell death and microvascular obstruction can be accurately assessed by MDCT (**Fig. 5**). MDCT infarct volume compared well with TTC staining (acute infarcts 21.1 $\pm$ 7.2% versus 20.4 $\pm$ 7.4%, mean difference 0.7%; chronic infarcts 4.15 $\pm$ 1.93% versus 4.92 $\pm$ 2.06%, mean difference 0.76%) and accurately reflected morphology and the transmural extent of injury in all animals.[56] Baks and colleagues[57] also reported that infarct size on delayed-enhanced CT using 10 pigs showed a good correlation with infarct size assessed with TTC pathology, and the correlation between delayed-enhanced CT and delayed-enhanced MRI in regards to infarct size was also good.

Mahnken and colleagues[58] compared both early-perfusion deficits and delayed-enhanced MDCT to delayed-enhanced MRI in a group of 28 patients after reperfusion of an acute myocardial infarction. Delayed-enhanced MDCT performed 15 minutes after contrast injection was shown to be more accurate than early-enhanced MDCT when compared with MRI in detecting both infarct size and location. While delayed-enhanced MDCT slightly overestimated infarct size, early enhancement significantly underestimated infarct size. Choe and colleagues[53] showed that there was a small, but statistically significant difference in

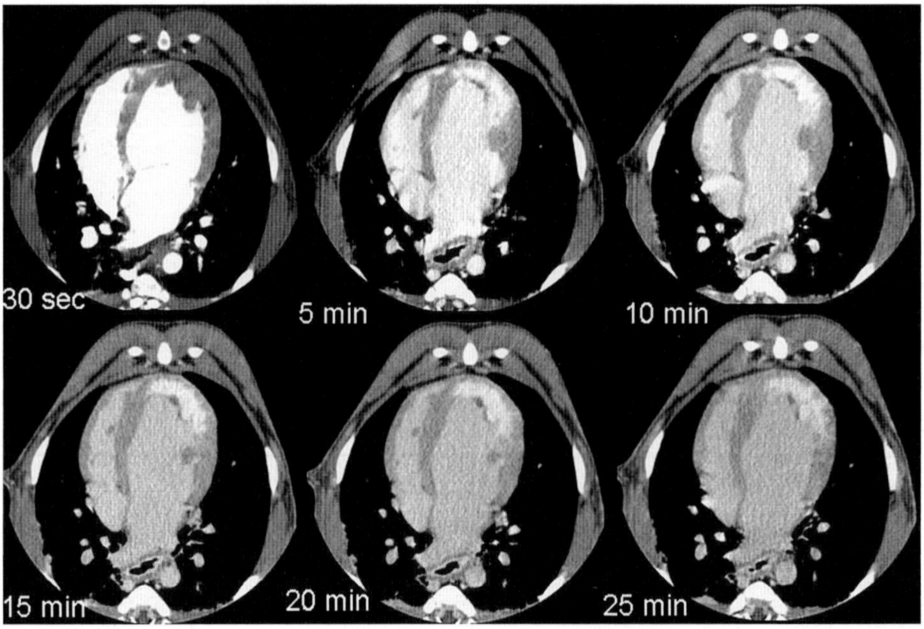


**Fig. 5.** Axial temporal image series demonstrating postreperfusion contrast agent kinetics after 150-mL injection of contrast. The signal density of the infarct in the first pass is substantially lower than that of the remote myocardium and indicates subendocardial microvascular obstruction. Five minutes after injection, the signal density of the damaged myocardial region is significantly greater than that of the remote normal myocardium and washes out over time. (*From* Lardo AC, Cordeiro MA, Silva C, et al. Contrast-enhanced multidetector computed tomography viability imaging after myocardial infarction: characterization of myocyte death, microvascular obstruction, and chronic scar. Circulation 2006;113(3):398; with permission.)

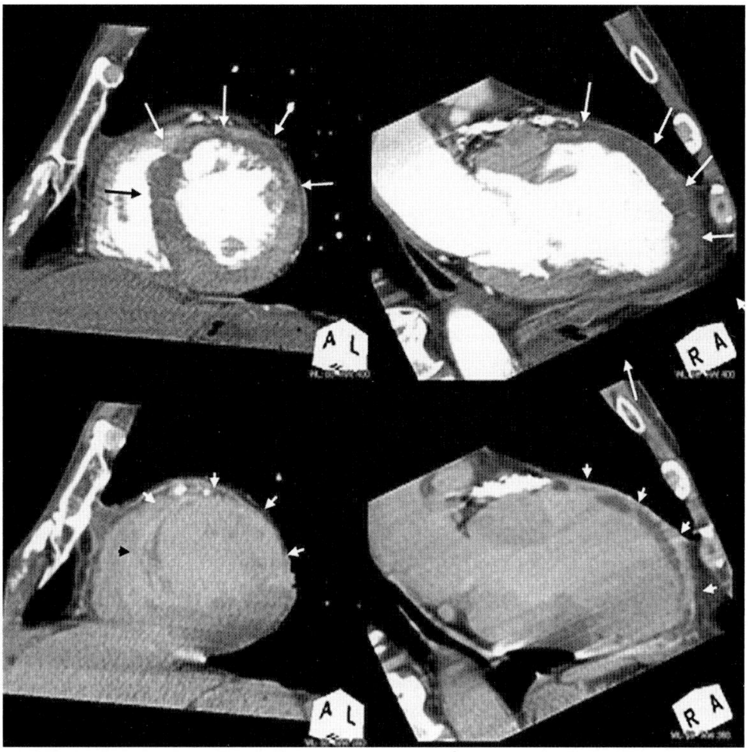


**Fig. 6.** Early first-pass perfusion CT and delayed-enhanced CT in a patient with chronic myocardial infarction. Rest first-pass perfusion MDCT shows wall thinning and hypo-enhanced area of anteroseptal, anterior, and anterolateral walls (*long arrows*). Delayed enhanced MDCT shows hyper-enhancement of these same walls with a large residual perfusion defect in same lesion (*short arrows*).

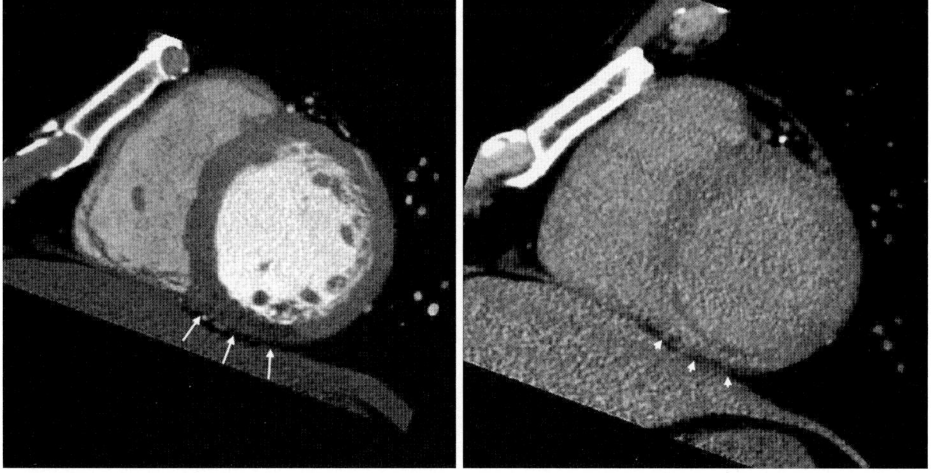

**Fig. 7.** Early first-pass perfusion CT and delayed-enhanced CT in the patient with acute myocardial infarction. Rest first-pass perfusion MDCT reveals hypo-enhancement of inferior wall (*long arrows*). Delayed-enhanced MDCT shows hyper-enhancement with residual subendocardial perfusion defect in the inferior wall (*short arrows*).

infarct size between the 5-minute delay MRI (25.9 ± 12.1%) and late CT (22.8 ± 11.8%) among 63 consecutive patients. Nieman and colleagues[52] reported that delayed hyper-enhancement was observed with MDCT at 11 of 15 examinations in which delayed enhancement was observed with delayed-enhanced MRI. Quantification of delayed hyper-enhancement had very good correlation between MDCT and cardiac MRI.

Koyama and colleagues[59] reported the utility of two-phase enhanced CT for the assessment of viability after reperfused acute myocardial infarction of 58 patients. The recovery of LVEF after intermediate periods (mean interval, 28 ± 4 days) was poorest in the patient group with early defect, delayed enhancement, and residual perfusion defect at 7 minutes (**Figs. 6** and **7**), and best in the patient group with delayed enhancement but no early defect or residual perfusion defect. Two-phase enhanced CT is useful in predicting LV functional recovery in patients who have had a reperfused acute myocardial infarction. Lessick and colleagues[60] also reported that in abnormal baseline segments, nonrecovery was clearly related to the presence and size of segment defect area for both early defect in first-pass perfusion and delayed-enhancement.

## SUMMARY

In conclusion, MDCT has the potential to evaluate cardiac function, myocardial perfusion, and viability. These capabilities, combined with the robust ability of MDCT to noninvasively image the coronary arteries, makes MDCT a comprehensive tool for the evaluation of coronary artery disease and its anatomic and physiologic impact on the myocardium. Recent technologic advances in MDCT technology in regards to detector coverage and spatial and temporal resolution are further advancing the capabilities of cardiac MDCT. Larger prospective clinical studies are required to further define the diagnostic role of MDCT.

## REFERENCES


1. Anno H, Katada K, Hasegawa H, et al. [Visualization of coronary arteries with helical scanning CT: diastolic reconstruction]. Nippon Igaku Hoshasen Gakkai Zasshi 1995;55(12):878–84 [in Japanese].
2. Achenbach S, Ulzheimer S, Baum U, et al. Noninvasive coronary angiography by retrospectively ECG-gated multislice spiral CT. Circulation 2000; 102(23):2823–8.
3. Cury RC, Nieman K, Shapiro MD, et al. Comprehensive assessment of myocardial perfusion defects, regional wall motion, and left ventricular function by using 64-section multidetector CT. Radiology 2008;248(2):466–75.
4. Tsai IC, Lee WL, Tsao CR, et al. Comprehensive evaluation of ischemic heart disease using MDCT. Am J Roentgenol 2008;191(1):64–72.
5. Mori S, Kondo C, Suzuki N, et al. Volumetric coronary angiography using the 256-detector row computed tomography scanner: comparison in vivo and in vitro with porcine models. Acta Radiol 2006;47:186–91.
6. Kondo C, Mori S, Endo M, et al. Real-time volumetric imaging of human heart without electrocardiographic gating by 256-detector row computed tomography: initial experience. J Comput Assist Tomogr 2005;29:694–8.
7. Hurlock GS, Higashino H, Mochizuki T. History of cardiac computed tomography: single to 320-detector row multislice computed tomography. Int J Cardiovasc Imaging 2009;25(1):31–42.
8. Schwarz F, Ruzsics B, Schoepf UJ, et al. Dual-energy CT of the heart—principles and protocols. Eur J Radiol 2008;68(3):423–33.
9. Kalra MK, Brady TJ. Current status and future directions in technical developments of cardiac computed tomography. J Cardiovasc Comput Tomogr 2008;2(2):71–80.
10. Mahnken AH, Muhlenbruch G, Koos R, et al. Automated vs. manual assessment of left ventricular function in cardiac multidetector row computed tomography: comparison with magnetic resonance imaging. Eur Radiol 2006;16(7):1416–23.
11. Mahnken AH, Koos R, Katoh M, et al. Sixteen-slice spiral CT versus MR imaging for the assessment of left ventricular function in acute myocardial infarction. Eur Radiol 2005;15:714–20.
12. Dewey M, Muller M, Teige F, et al. Evaluation of a semiautomatic software tool for left ventricular function analysis with 16-slice computed tomography. Eur Radiol 2006;16:25–31.
13. Belge B, Coche E, Pasquet A, et al. Accurate estimation of global and regional cardiac function by retrospectively gated multidetector row computed tomography: comparison with cine magnetic resonance imaging. Eur Radiol 2006;16(7):1424–33.
14. Schlosser T, Mohrs OK, Magedanz A, et al. Assessment of left ventricular function and mass in patients undergoing computed tomography (CT) coronary angiography using 64-detector-row CT: comparison to magnetic resonance imaging. Acta Radiol 2007; 48:30–5.
15. van der Vleuten PA, Willems TP, Gotte MJ, et al. Quantification of global left ventricular function: comparison of multidetector computed tomography and magnetic resonance imaging. A meta-analysis and review of the current literature. Acta Radiol 2006;47(10):1049–57.

16. Sugeng L, Mor-Avi V, Weinert L, et al. Quantitative assessment of left ventricular size and function -side-by-side comparison of real-time three-dimensional echocardiography and computed tomography with magnetic resonance reference. Circulation 2006; 114:654–61.
17. Juergens KU, Seifarth H, David Maintz, et al. MDCT determination of volume and function of the left ventricle: are short-axis image reformation necessary? Am J Roentgenol 2006;186:S371–8.
18. Kim TH, Ryu YH, Hur J, et al. Evaluation of right ventricular volume and mass using retrospective ECG-gated cardiac multidetector computed tomography: comparison with first-pass radionuclide angiography. Eur Radiol 2005;15(9):1987–93.
19. Stolzmann P, Scheffel H, Leschka S, et al. Reference values for quantitative left ventricular and left atrial measurements in cardiac computed tomography. Eur Radiol 2008;18(8):1625–34.
20. Mahnken AH, Hohl C, Suess C, et al. Influence of heart rate and temporal resolution on left-ventricular volumes in cardiac multislice spiral computed tomography. A phantom study. Invest Radiol 2006;41:429–35.
21. Mahnken AH, Bruder H, Suess C, et al. Dual-source computed tomography for assessing cardiac function. A phantom study. Invest Radiol 2007;42:491–8.
22. Brodoefel H, Kramer U, Reimann A, et al. Dual-source CT with improved temporal resolution in assessment of left ventricular function: a pilot study. Am J Roentgenol 2007;189:1064–70.
23. Bastarrika G, Arraiza M, De Cecco CN, et al. Quantification of left ventricular function and mass in heart transplant recipients using dual-source CT and MRI: initial clinical experience. Eur Radiol 2008;18:1784–90.
24. Busch S, Johnson TR, Wintersperger BJ, et al. Quantitative assessment of left ventricular function with dual-source CT in comparison to cardiac magnetic resonance imaging: initial findings. Eur Radiol 2008;18(3):570–5.
25. Hachamovitch R, Hayes SW, Friedman JD, et al. Comparison of the short-term survival benefit associated with revascularization compared with medical therapy in patients with no prior coronary artery disease undergoing stress myocardial perfusion single photon emission computed tomography. Circulation 2003;107(23):2900–7.
26. Rispler S, Keidar Z, Ghersin E, et al. Integrated single-photon emission computed tomography and computed tomography coronary angiography for the assessment of hemodynamically significant coronary artery lesions. J Am Coll Cardiol 2007; 49(10):1059–67.
27. Di Carli MF, Dorbala S, Hachamovitch R. Integrated cardiac PET-CT for the diagnosis and management of CAD. J Nucl Cardiol 2006;13(2):139–44.
28. Naito H, Hamada S, Takamiya M, et al. Significance of dipyridamole loading in ultrafast X-ray computed tomography for detection of myocardial ischemia. Invest Radiol 1995;30:389–95.
29. Knollmann FD, Muschick P, Krause W, et al. Detection of myocardial ischemia by electron beam CT. Acta Radiol 2001;42:386–92.
30. Rumberger JA, Feiring AJ, Lipton MJ, et al. Use of ultrafast computed tomography to quantitate regional myocardial perfusion a preliminary report. J Am Coll Cardiol 1987;9:57–69.
31. Wolfkiel CJ, Ferguson JL, Chomka EV, et al. Measurement of myocardial blood flow by ultrafast computed tomography. Circulation 1987;76(6): 1262–73.
32. George RT, Jerosch-Herold M, Silva C, et al. Quantification of myocardial perfusion using dynamic 64-detector computed tomography. Invest Radiol 2007;42:815–22.
33. Daghini E, Primak AN, Chade AR, et al. Evaluation of porcine myocardial microvascular permeability and fractional vascular volume using 64-slice helical computed tomography (CT). Invest Radiol 2007; 42(5):274–82.
34. George RT, Lardo AC, Lima JAC. Computed tomography for the assessment of myocardial perfusion. In: Gerber TC, editor. Computed tomography of the cardiovascular system. London: Informa; 2007. p. 441–8.
35. Kurata A, Mochizuki T, Koyama Y, et al. Myocardial perfusion imaging using adenosine triphosphate stress multi-slice spiral computed tomography alternative to stress myocardial perfusion scintigraphy. Circ J 2005;69(5):550–7.
36. George R, Silva C, Cordeiro MA, et al. Multidetector computed tomography myocardial perfusion imaging during adenosine stress. J Am Coll Cardiol 2006;48: 153–60.
37. George RT, Arbab-Zadeh A, Miller JM, et al. Adenosine stress 64 and 256 row detector computed tomography angiography and perfusion imaging: a pilot study evaluating the transmural extent of perfusion abnormalities to predict atherosclerosis causing myocardial ischemia. Circ Cardiovasc Imaging 2009;2:174–82.
38. Groves AM, Goh V, Rajasekharan S, et al. CT coronary angiography: quantitative assessment of myocardial perfusion using test bolus data-initial experience. Eur Radiol 2008;18:2155–63.
39. George RT, Kitagawa K, Laws K, et al. Combined adenosine stress perfusion and coronary angiography using 320-row detector dynamic volume computed tomography in patients with suspected coronary artery disease. Circulation 2008;118: S936.
40. George RT, Kitagawa K, Lautamaki R, et al. Adenosine Stress myocardial perfusion imaging using 256-row dynamic volume computed tomography. Circulation 2008;118:S936.

41. Wu KC, Lima JA. Noninvasive imaging of myocardial viability: current techniques and future developments. Circ Res 2003;93(12):1146–58.
42. Thomson LE, Kim RJ, Judd RM. Magnetic resonance imaging for the assessment of myocardial viability. J Magn Reson Imaging 2004;19(6): 771–88.
43. Cerqueira MD, Jacobson AF. Assessment of myocardial viability with SPECT and PET imaging. Am J Roentgenol 1989;153(3):477–83.
44. Stillman AE, Wilke N, Jerosch-Herold M. Myocardial viability. Radiol Clin North Am 1999;37(2):361–78.
45. Newhouse JH. Fluid compartment distribution of intravenous iothalamate in the dog. Invest Radiol 1977;12(4):364–7.
46. Newhouse JH, Murphy RX Jr. Tissue distribution of soluble contrast: effect of dose variation and changes with time. Am J Roentgenol 1981;136(3): 463–7.
47. Canty JM Jr, Judd RM, Brody AS, et al. First-pass entry of nonionic contrast agent into the myocardial extravascular space. Effects on radiographic estimates of transit time and blood volume. Circulation 1991;84(5):2071–8.
48. Schuleri KH, Centola M, George RT, et al. Characterization of peri-infarct zone heterogeneity by contrast enhanced multi-detector computed tomography. J Am Coll Cardiol 2009;53(18):1699–707.
49. Nikolaou K, Knez A, Sagmeister S, et al. Assessment of myocardial infarctions using multidetector-row computed tomography. J Comput Assist Tomogr 2004;28(2):286–92.
50. Hoffmann U, Millea R, Enzweiler C, et al. Acute myocardial infarction: contrast-enhanced multidetector row CT in a porcine model. Radiology 2004;231(3):697–701.
51. Nikolaou K, Sanz J, Poon M, et al. Assessment of myocardial perfusion and viability from routine contrast-enhanced 16-detector-row computed tomography of the heart: preliminary results. Eur Radiol 2005;15(5):864–71.
52. Nieman K, Shapiro MD, Ferencik M, et al. Reperfused myocardial infarction: contrast-enhanced 64-Section CT in comparison to MR imaging. Radiology 2008;247(1):49–56.
53. Choe YH, Choo KS, Jeon ES, et al. Comparison of MDCT and MRI in the detection and sizing of acute and chronic myocardial infarcts. Eur J Radiol 2008; 66(2):292–9.
54. Wada H, Kobayashi Y, Yasu T, et al. Multi-detector computed tomography for imaging of subendocardial infarction prediction of wall motion recovery after reperfused anterior myocardial infarction. Circ J 2004;68:512–4.
55. Ingkanisorn WP, Rhoads KL, Aletras AH, et al. Gadolinium delayed enhancement cardiovascular magnetic resonance correlates with clinical measures of myocardial infarction. J Am Coll Cardiol 2004; 43(12):2253–9.
56. Lardo AC, Cordeiro MA, Silva C, et al. Contrast-enhanced multidetector computed tomography viability imaging after myocardial infarction: characterization of myocyte death, microvascular obstruction, and chronic scar. Circulation 2006;113(3): 394–404.
57. Baks T, Cademartiri F, Moelker AD, et al. Multislice computed tomography and magnetic resonance imaging for the assessment of reperfused acute myocardial infarction. J Am Coll Cardiol 2006; 48(1):144–52.
58. Mahaken AH, Muhlenbruch G, Gunther RW, et al. CT imaging of myocardial viability experimental and clinical evidence. Cardiovasc J Afr 2007;18(3):169–74.
59. Koyama Y, Matsuoka H, Mochizuki T, et al. Assessment of reperfused acute myocardial infarction with two-phase contrast-enhanced helical CT prediction of left ventricular function and wall thickness. Radiology 2005;235(3):804–11.
60. Lessick J, Dragu R, Mutlak D, et al. Is functional improvement after myocardial infarction predicted with myocardial enhancement patterns at multidetector CT? Radiology 2007;244(3):736–44.

# Recent Technologic Advances in Multi-Detector Row Cardiac CT

Sandra Simon Halliburton, PhD

**KEYWORDS**

- Computed tomography • Radiation dose
- Temporal resolution • Spatial resolution
- Scan time • Tissue differentiation

Ever since its inception, there has been a desire to apply x-ray CT to imaging of the cardiovascular system. Early CT, however, lacked many technical capabilities required for imaging of the heart.

Data acquisition with conventional CT technology is accomplished by mechanically rotating an x-ray tube and detector array around the patient. The slow rotational speed of early equipment required 300 seconds for the acquisition of enough data to reconstruct a single image.[1] With significant improvements between 1972 and 1990,[2] this time was reduced to 2 seconds but was still too long for cardiac imaging. Additionally, data could only be acquired in the axial (ie, sequential or step-and-shoot) mode with limited longitudinal or *z*-coverage per rotation, resulting in very long scan times.

In 1983, electron beam CT technology was introduced.[3] With this technology, an electron beam, rather than an x-ray tube, is rotated around the patient. X-rays are produced when the rotating electron beam strikes a tungsten target encircling the patient. Attenuated x-rays were measured by a stationary detector. This technology, then, eliminated the requirement for mechanical motion of an x-ray tube/detector system around the patient and reduced the acquisition time for each axial image to 50 to 100 milliseconds. Although the temporal resolution of electron beam CT was sufficient for cardiac imaging, long scan times, poor spatial resolution, and lack of x-ray power limited clinical application.

Parallel advances in conventional CT included, most notably, the introduction of helical (ie, spiral) scanning in 1989.[4,5] Although significant improvements in volume coverage speed were realized, 1 second was still needed to acquire enough projection data to reconstruct a single image, prohibiting diagnostic imaging of the heart.

The advent of systems with sub-second rotation times and ECG-synchronized scanning in 1994 brought conventional CT into the domain of cardiac imaging. Initial results demonstrated the clinical potential of conventional CT, but technical restrictions still limited cardiac applications primarily to coronary artery calcium scoring.[6,7]

Conventional CT did not have a major impact on cardiac imaging until the introduction of multidetector row CT (MDCT) scanners in 1998,[8,9] permitting the simultaneous acquisition of four slices, rotation times as short as 500 milliseconds, images as thin as 1.25 mm, and scan times for coverage of the entire heart equal to 35 to 40 seconds. Further improvements were observed with the introduction of 8-slice scanners in 2001, 16-slice in 2002,[10,11] 64-slice in 2004,[12] dual-source scanners in 2006,[13] and 320-slice scanner in 2007.[14] This evolution of MDCT scanners has

S.S. Halliburton is the recipient of a research grant from Siemens Medical Solutions, Healthcare Sector Imaging and IT Division.

Imaging Institute, Cardiovascular Imaging, Cleveland Clinic, 9500 Euclid Avenue/J1-222, Cleveland, OH 44195, USA

*E-mail address:* hallibs@ccf.org

Cardiol Clin 27 (2009) 655–664
doi:10.1016/j.ccl.2009.06.007
0733-8651/09/$ – see front matter 

resulted in not only an increased number of slices per rotation, but also rotation times as short as 270 milliseconds, images as thin as 0.5 mm, and scan times for the whole heart ranging from less than 1 second to 10 seconds.[13,14]

Despite the significant technical advances that have spurred the widespread application of CT to clinical cardiovascular imaging, efforts are still being made to further reduce radiation dose, improve temporal and spatial resolution, decrease scan time, and improve tissue differentiation. This article discusses the recent technical advances resulting from these efforts.

## RADIATION DOSE

Amid reports of increased radiation exposure to the public from medical imaging,[15] namely CT, and growing concerns about the associated biologic risk,[16,17] CT scanner manufacturers are aggressively pursuing radiation-exposure reduction techniques. One new feature, adaptive prepatient *z*-collimation, is designed to reduce radiation exposure by preventing x-rays not contributing data to image formation from reaching the patient, and is applied by default with the selection of the scan protocol. Other strategies modify the x-ray tube current in real time according to user-defined variables, thereby decreasing the number of x-ray photons interacting with the patient. Still another strategy, the use of noise-reducing reconstruction algorithms, approaches dose reduction indirectly through improved use of the attenuation data.

### *Pre-patient Z-collimation*

As the total collimated detector width in *z* increases (associated with an increased number of detector rows), the number of x-rays passing outside the planned scan length and not contributing to image formation increases.[18] Adaptive prepatient *z*-collimators were recently introduced on some CT systems to reduce x-ray exposure by restricting the divergent x-ray beam along the *z*-axis and preventing x-rays outside the planned scan length from reaching the patient (**Fig. 1**). The amount by which the scan length actually exposed to x-rays exceeds the planned scan length is termed "*z*-overscanning," or overranging. *Z*-overscanning can occur with either helical or axial imaging.

In the helical scan mode, reconstruction algorithms require extra rotations of the x-ray source outside the desired scan length to obtain sufficient data for image reconstruction at the start and end.[2] X-ray attenuation data generated from these extra rotations do not provide images at table positions outside the planned scan length. A reduction in *z*-overscanning with helical imaging can be achieved using a dynamic prepatient *z*-collimator.[19] Opposing collimator blades automatically open at the start of helical data acquisition and close at the end of acquisition to block radiation not contributing to image formation.

In the axial scan mode, *z*-overscanning occurs when the desired scan length is not an integer multiple of the total *z*-collimated detector width. Although differences between the planned scan length and the exposed scan length are relatively

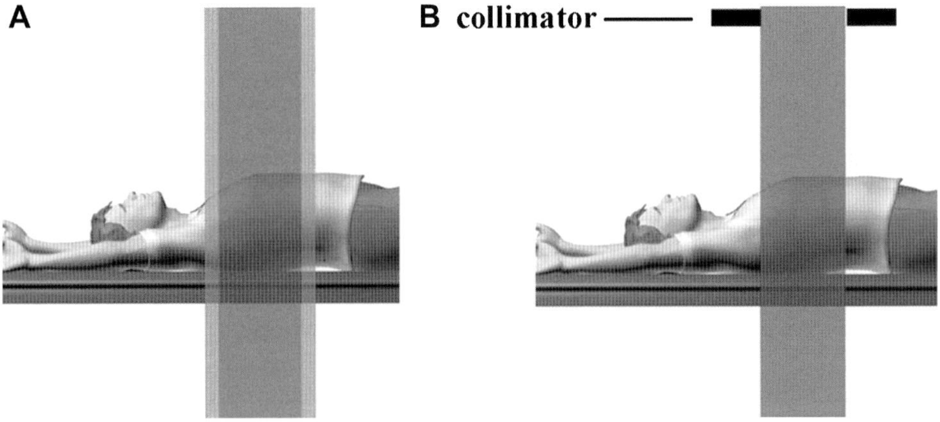


**Fig. 1.** Side-view of patient imaged (*A*) without (*B*) and with prepatient *z*-collimation. During scanning, some x-rays pass outside the planned scan length and do not contribute data to image formation (*z*-overscanning). Without prepatient collimation (*A*), this results in patient exposure to unnecessary radiation (light red). With prepatient collimation, only the desired anatomy is exposed (dark red) and z-overscanning is minimized. Note: the actual extent of *z*-overscanning depends on the scan mode (helical or axial) and the total *z*-detector width.

small, with a narrow total z-axis collimated-detector width, these differences can become significant with increasing z-axis detector coverage and constitute a major source of unnecessary x-ray exposure. One approach to reducing z-overscanning for axial imaging is to provide a set of automatically selectable z-detector collimations with a range of total widths to more precisely match the total z-collimated detector width to many different scan ranges.[19]

## *ECG-based X-ray Tube-current Modulation*

Recent advances in the prospectively ECG-triggered axial technique have allowed application to imaging of the coronary arteries.[20–23] With this technique, the x-ray tube current is switched on only during the desired cardiac phase, significantly limiting x-ray exposure. Appropriate timing of data acquisition relies on accurate estimates of the expected length of the upcoming RR interval. Therefore, the main disadvantage of prospectively ECG-triggered axial data acquisition is vulnerability to cardiac motion artifacts in patients with irregular heart rates. Technical developments aimed at minimizing cardiac motion artifacts with axial imaging include collection of additional data beyond the minimum required for image reconstruction (ie, padding) to permit minor retrospective adjustments of the reconstruction window. It is important to note, however, that this approach significantly increases x-ray exposure. In addition, many manufacturers have recently introduced automated arrhythmia-rejection methods that postpone axial data acquisition, if an irregularity is detected, until the heart rate stabilizes.

Despite the significant advances in axial imaging, retrospective ECG-gated helical data acquisition is still preferred for patients with high or irregular heart rates. With this technique, the x-ray tube current is switched on during the entire scan. The ECG signal is recorded during data acquisition and used to retrospectively gate data reconstruction to one or more desired cardiac phases. Retrospective referencing of the ECG signal now allows the deletion of extra systolic beats, the insertion of missed beats, and the shifting of R-peak locations to adjust for arrhythmia on most CT systems. Retrospectively, ECG-gated helical techniques are then less sensitive to heart-rate irregularities than axial techniques.

ECG-based tube-current modulation is employed with helical data acquisition to significantly decrease x-ray exposure (**Fig. 2**). The tube current is at a maximum only during the cardiac phase of interest and is reduced substantially outside this phase. Although data are available during the

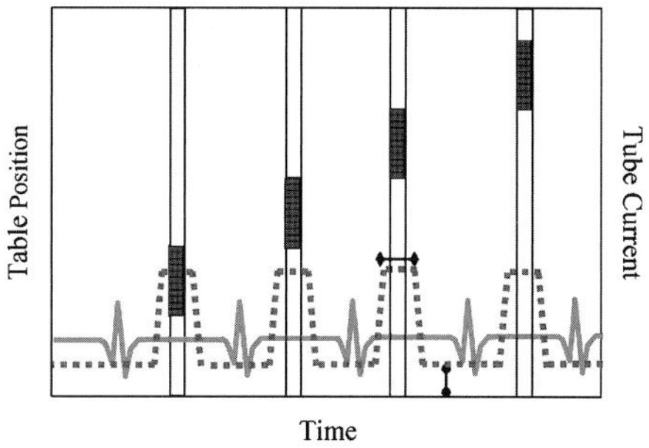


**Fig. 2.** Basic helical technique for cardiac imaging with ECG-based prospective on-line modulation of the tube current. Data are acquired continuously during movement of the patient table. Tube current (*dotted line*) is at a maximum during imaging of the desired cardiac phase or phases but is reduced outside this region. Some CT scanners permit adjustment of the duration of maximum tube current (*double-headed diamond line*) as well as the magnitude of the minimum tube current (*double-headed circle line*). Data are retrospectively referenced to the ECG-signal (*solid line*) and reconstructed at the desired time points. Vertical rectangles indicate reconstruction periods. Small horizontal rectangles indicate reconstructed images.

entire cardiac cycle, image quality during periods of low current is limited. User selection of the minimum tube current (eg, 20% versus 4% of maximum tube current) was recently introduced to permit additional dose savings in many clinical situations.[24]

ECG-based tube-current modulation, however, imposes limitations on helical imaging of patients with irregular heart rates. Because tube-current modulation is prescribed before scanning, changes in heart rate could result in unintended lowering of the tube current during a desired phase of reconstruction for a given cardiac cycle. For this reason, ECG-based tube-current modulation is often not used with helical imaging for such patients, resulting in very high radiation doses.[25]

Several manufacturers have recently developed new strategies for ECG-based tube-current modulation with helical imaging, increasing the robustness of the technique for patients with irregular heart rates. One strategy is to allow user adjustment of the maximum tube-current duration before scanning; rather than restricting the user to two discrete choices—maximum tube current during one phase of the cardiac cycle or maximum tube current during the entire cardiac cycle—the user is given the flexibility to apply the maximum tube current over a continuous range. A second strategy, aimed at improving the utility of ECG-based tube-current modulation for patients with severe arrhythmia, is the temporary or permanent suspension of tube-current modulation if beat-to-beat variation exceeds a threshold value during data acquisition. In this case, the risk of improperly timed downward modulation of the tube current is virtually eliminated. Although radiation exposure with respect to traditional approaches to ECG-based tube-current modulation is increased with both strategies, exposure is still less than if ECG-based tube-current modulation is not used.[24]

### *Anatomic-based Tube-current Modulation*

The x-ray tube current can also be modulated automatically according to patient anatomy to reduce radiation exposure. The tube current can be modulated along the *x*-, *y*-, and *z*-directions during scanning based on local tissue thickness determined from scout imaging without sacrificing image noise.[26] Tube current is reduced at projection angles and table positions requiring less x-ray penetration. This approach can yield dose savings with axial imaging but interferes with ECG-based modulation and, therefore, has limited application to helical imaging. In practice, ECG-based tube-current modulation is given priority during helical imaging and anatomic-based modulation serves only to determine the optimal nominal tube current necessary to achieve the desired noise based on patient attenuation in the scout image. Although anatomic-based tube-current modulation is well-established, cardiac applications have not benefited from the technique because of the dominance of helical imaging. The recent shift toward axial imaging, however, should mean increased use of anatomic-based tube-current modulation and further reduction in cardiac CT dose.

### *High Pitch*

A low-beam pitch (eg, 0.2) is typically required for helical acquisition of cardiac data because a pitch too high for the patient's heart rate results in the table moving too far between consecutive cardiac cycles and gaps in the acquired data. This is of particular concern for multisegment reconstruction algorithms that use data from two or more consecutive cardiac cycles (rather than a single cardiac cycle) to reconstruct each image.

The high temporal resolution afforded by existing dual source CT (DSCT) technology for cardiac imaging permits single-segment reconstruction and heart rate-dependent pitch. Higher pitch values (eg, 0.2–0.5) can be used with higher heart rates to achieve significant dose savings.[27]

A new application of DSCT technology permits ECG-referenced helical scanning at very high pitch values. By interleaving data measured from two detector systems separated by 90°, pitch can be increased up to 3.2 within the limited scan field-of-view covered by both detectors.[28] Helical scanning with such high pitch values reduces the amount of redundant data collected substantially decreasing radiation exposure.

### *Reconstruction Algorithms*

One option for decreasing x-ray exposure is the use of noise-reducing statistical iterative reconstruction algorithms (**Fig. 3**).[29] Iterative reconstruction algorithms were used with the first CT

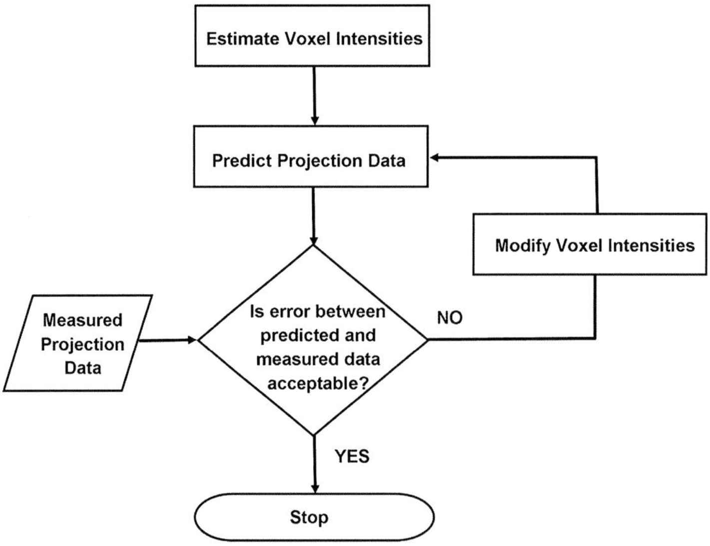


**Fig. 3.** Flow chart diagramming the basic steps of iterative reconstruction.

scanners but were soon rejected as the standard for CT image reconstruction in favor of faster, less computationally intensive filtered back-projection techniques. Iterative reconstruction algorithms assume initial attenuation coefficients for all voxels and use these coefficients to predict projection data. Predicted projection data are compared with actual, measured projection data and voxel attenuations are modified until the error between estimated and measured projection data is acceptable. Compared with standard analytical reconstruction methods based on filtered back-projections, statistical iterative reconstruction produces equivalent signal-to-noise ratios (SNRs) at lower radiation doses without a loss in spatial resolution.[29,30] Recent advances in computer-processing hardware and the increased efficiency of new iterative reconstruction algorithms[29,30] have sparked the reemergence of these algorithms as an option for CT image reconstruction.

## TEMPORAL RESOLUTION

The term "temporal resolution" is used in CT imaging to describe the time needed to acquire enough data for reconstruction of a single image. The temporal resolution needs to be sufficiently high for cardiac imaging to limit cardiac motion artifacts. Because approximately 180° of projection data are required by cardiac algorithms to reconstruct an image for a sufficiently small, centered object, the temporal resolution is approximated as one-half the gantry rotation time for single x-ray source CT scanners and one-fourth the gantry rotation time for dual x-ray source scanners. Temporal resolution has significantly improved from 250 to 400 milliseconds with early MDCT systems, to 75 to 175 milliseconds with state-of-the-art systems as a result of faster gantry rotation times and inclusion of a second x-ray source/detector system.

### Gantry Rotation

The gantry rotation time is the time required for the x-ray tube/detector system to rotate 360° around the patient. Faster gantry rotation means faster acquisition of the data needed to reconstruct each image and, subsequently, improved temporal resolution. Values for state-of-the-art scanners range from 270 to 350 milliseconds.

Even faster gantry rotation is desired but limited in part by the mechanical forces (eg, centrifugal forces and frictional forces) acting on the system. One manufacturer recently overcame some of the mechanical limitations by developing an air-bearing rotator design that reduces friction and allows faster gantry rotation (270 milliseconds). Faster gantry rotation is also limited by requirements on x-ray tube power. As rotation times shorten it is necessary to increase the x-ray tube current to maintain x-ray flux and achieve the desired SNR. Although faster gantry rotations have been possible recently because of augmented x-ray power, increased demands on gantry rotation would stretch tube power beyond current limits.[31] Finally, a third obstacle to faster gantry rotation is the data transfer rate.

### Number of X-ray Sources

An alternative approach for improving temporal resolution is the addition of a second measurement system within the gantry. A commercial DSCT system was recently introduced employing two x-ray sources mounted opposite two detector arrays and separated by 90°. The two x-ray source/detector systems rotate together once every 330 milliseconds and collect the data needed to reconstruct an image in 83 milliseconds. This approach has obvious advantages for cardiac imaging, given the significant gains in temporal resolution. A challenge facing dual-source compared with single-source CT with the same *z* coverage is additional cross-scattered x-ray radiation, resulting in increased Hounsfield Unit magnitude of common streak and cupping artifacts and increased noise. Phantom work has shown that artifacts can be reduced by applying scatter-correction algorithms and noise can be restored with additional x-ray doses.[32] Clinical studies have demonstrated, however, that dose-saving features of commercially available DSCT systems counter the dose cost resulting in images of the coronary arteries, with improved image quality and decreased noise without an increase in radiation dose, compared with single-source CT.[24] Further improvements in temporal resolution can be achieved with additional sources (ie, greater than two) but technical realization is not forthcoming.

## SPATIAL RESOLUTION

Improved spatial resolution remains a priority for cardiac CT. The limits of spatial resolution are dictated by scanner geometry, x-ray focus size, aperture and movement during measurement, and detector element size and spacing.[2] No significant improvement in in-plane (*x*–*y* plane) spatial resolution has been realized with newer compared with older MDCT scanners. However, considerable progress in through-plane (*z*-axis) resolution has been achieved during the evolution of MDCT, primarily because of the availability of thinner collimated detector widths. Early MDCT scanners provided approximately 1-mm collimated detector widths for routine cardiac scanning, but state-of-the-art systems provide 0.5-mm to 0.625-mm widths. Further improvement in through-plane spatial resolution has been achieved at these collimated detector widths on several newer MDCT systems with the implementation of *z*-flying x-ray focal-spot techniques.

With the recent enhancement in *z* resolution, isotropic spatial resolution can be achieved for cardiac CT, typically of $0.5 \times 0.5 \times 0.5$ mm$^2$. Because improvement in spatial resolution is associated with an increase in image noise (fewer x-ray photons reach thinner detectors), further improvement requires an increase in x-ray exposure beyond acceptable levels, an increase in detector efficiency through the development of new detector materials or better detector electronics, or implementation of noise-reducing reconstruction algorithms.

### *Z-flying X-ray Focal Spot*

Deflection of the focal spot, or the idealized point on the surface of the x-ray tube anode from which x-rays emerge in the *x-y* plane, has long been used to double the number of samples acquired across the field-of-view and improve in-plane spatial resolution.[2] More recently, several manufacturers have implemented x-ray focal spot deflection along the *z*-axis, such that two consecutive measurements are shifted by an amount equal to half of the collimated detector slice width. Two interleaved readings are then acquired with twice the number of measured values in the *z*-direction and at half the sampling distance (**Fig. 4**), compared with acquisition of a single reading per rotation. Using this technique, the theoretical limit of through-plane resolution for 0.6-mm collimated detector widths can be improved to 0.4 mm.[12]

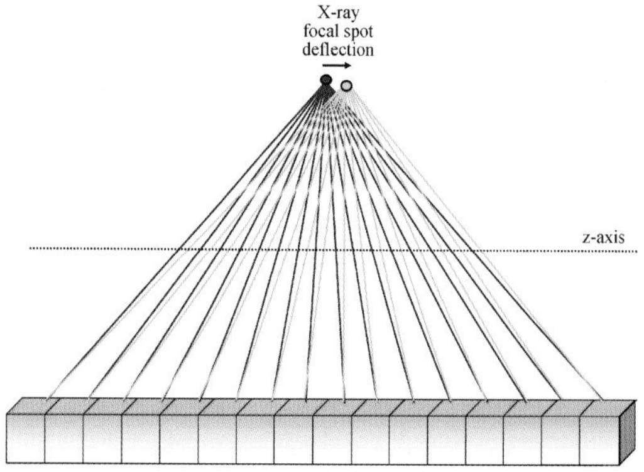


**Fig. 4.** Deflection of x-ray focal spot along *z*-axis. Two consecutive measurements are shifted by an amount equal to half the collimated detector slice width. Two interleaved readings are acquired with twice the number of measured values in the *z*-direction and at half the sampling distance compared with acquisition of a single reading.

### *Detector Composition*

CT systems employ solid-state detectors to convert x-rays to digital signals. Incident x-rays are converted to visible light by a solid-state scintillator material. The visible light is detected by a photodiode and converted into an electrical signal. The development of scintillator material with improved detection efficiency or reduced afterglow might permit better spatial resolution without a noise penalty. Although a new detector material (Lutetium terbium aluminium garnet) was recently introduced for commercial use, it offers no improvements in detector efficiency and afterglow compared with existing materials used by other manufacturers (eg, gadolinium-oxide),[2] and thus, the material alone is unlikely to raise the industry standard for spatial resolution without a significant increase in radiation dose.

### *Reconstruction Algorithms*

Noise-reducing reconstruction algorithms, such as iterative reconstruction algorithms, offer the greatest potential for significant improvements in spatial resolution for cardiac CT. Iterative reconstruction algorithms can be used to provide images with equivalent SNR compared with filtered back-projection at lower radiation doses without a loss in spatial resolution, as described above or, alternatively, to provide SNR-equivalent images at the same radiation dose with improved spatial resolution.[29]

## SCAN TIME

The term "scan time" is used in CT to describe the time necessary to acquire all images in the scanned volume. Short scan times permit breath-holding during data acquisition and reduce the probability of respiratory motion artifacts. Extremely short scan times permit data acquisition during a single cardiac cycle and, additionally, reduce the likelihood of cardiac motion artifacts along the *z*-axis, such as banding or stair-step artifacts (incidence of cardiac motion artifacts in-plane is dictated by temporal resolution). Among the most dramatic changes in CT during the last decade, impacting cardiovascular imaging, is the decrease in scan time. The scan time for coronary imaging decreased from approximately 35 to 40 seconds with early MDCT scanners to less than 1 second with some state-of-the-art systems.[14,28]

This leap was accomplished primarily by increasing z-coverage per rotation through the design of detector arrays with increasing numbers of detector rows, and by enabling very high pitch data acquisition through the simultaneous use of two x-ray sources.

### Wide Multidetector Arrays

Increased z-coverage per rotation and, subsequently, decreased scan time, is associated with a greater number of detector rows in a multidetector array. It is important to note that the number of detector rows does not necessarily equal the number of slices that can be acquired per rotation; some scanners sample each detector twice per rotation (using the z-flying focal-spot technique described above), such that the number of slices acquired per rotation is two times the number of detector rows used. Z-coverage per rotation at the isocenter varies significantly across recently introduced scanners; new 128-slice scanners from two manufacturers sample 64 detector rows with 0.6-mm slice collimation twice, yielding 3.8 cm of z-coverage per rotation,[31] a new 256-slice model samples 128 detector rows with 0.625-mm slice collimation twice, achieving 8 cm of z-coverage during one rotation,[19] and a 320-detector row system with 0.5-mm slice collimation provides 16 cm of z-coverage per rotation, sampling the detectors only once.[14] Scan times on these new systems for coronary imaging range from less than 5 seconds[22] to less than 1 second.[14,31] The 320-detector row system requires only one rotation to image the heart for low heart rates, so total scan time is approximately equal to the temporal resolution at the isocenter or 175 milliseconds.

One of the greatest challenges facing CT imaging with wide multidetector arrays is the transition from fan-beam to cone-beam geometry and the implications for image reconstruction. New reconstruction algorithms were recently developed, enabling accurate reconstruction of cone-beam data.[33] In addition, like DSCT scanning, scanning with wide multidetector arrays faces challenges stemming from scattered radiation. X-ray scatter for a DSCT system is comparable to a single-source system with twice the z-coverage.[32,34] Early results indicate that these barriers to wide-multidetector array imaging have been largely overcome with the recently introduced clinical systems.[14,19,35]

### High Pitch

As described above, new DSCT technology permits gapless z-sampling during helical cardiac imaging at extremely high pitch values. The technology offers 0.28-second gantry rotation time and approximately 4-cm z-coverage per rotation, such that helical imaging with a pitch of 3.2 results in 43 cm per second scan speed.[31] Therefore, typical cardiac ranges can be scanned in less than 0.3 seconds, confining helical data acquisition to a single heart beat (for patients with low heart rates) (**Fig. 5**).

## TISSUE DIFFERENTIATION

Although CT currently provides good differentiation of tissues, there is a desire to push the technology further. Each pixel, or picture element, in the CT image corresponds to a three-dimensional voxel, or volume element, within the patient. Each image pixel displays a tissue attenuation coefficient describing the average attenuation of x-rays within each corresponding patient voxel. Tissue-attenuation coefficients depend on the composition and density of the tissue within the voxel, as well as the x-ray photon energy.

X-rays at energies within the diagnostic imaging range primarily interact with matter via Compton scattering and the photoelectric effect. Photoelectric emissions dominate at lower x-ray energy levels and depend heavily on the atomic number of the material, while Compton scatter dominates at higher energies and is more dependent on the density of the material.[36] Therefore, different

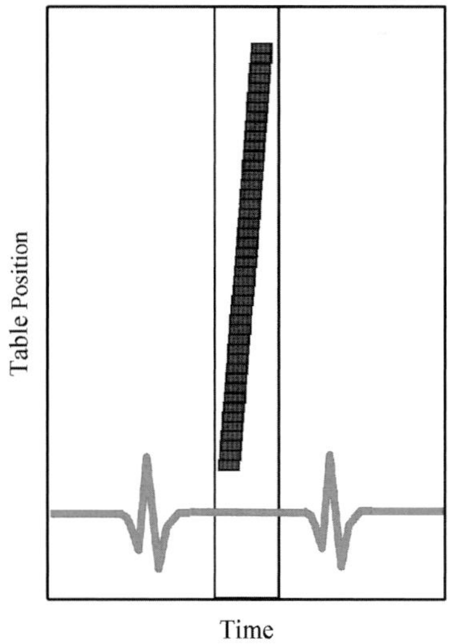


**Fig. 5.** Helical technique for cardiac imaging with very high pitch. Data are acquired continuously during movement of the patient table. Data acquisition is triggered by the ECG signal (*solid line*) and completed during a single cardiac cycle. Vertical rectangle indicates acquisition period. Small horizontal rectangles indicate reconstructed images.

attenuation values are observed for the same material at different x-ray energies.

CT imaging typically relies on one set of attenuation data obtained using a broad x-ray spectrum, with energies ranging from 20 keV to 150 keV, depending on the peak voltage applied across the x-ray tube. Dual-energy imaging describes the acquisition of two spectrally distinct attenuation data sets and has been studied since the late 1970s[36,37] as a potential tool for improved tissue discrimination with CT. Significant resources have recently been devoted to providing dual-energy techniques on clinical CT systems.

One approach to dual-energy imaging is the use of two x-ray tubes to simultaneously apply two x-ray spectra, each generated using a different peak x-ray tube voltage (eg, 80 kVp and 140 kVp), and therefore spanning different energy ranges. Two data sets with differing attenuation characteristics are then obtained from the region of interest. Dual-energy techniques using this approach are commercially available and have already been applied to imaging of the heart.[38,39] Although promising, the ability to discriminate certain tissues is limited by the overlap of attenuation data, resulting at least in part from overlap of the low- and high-energy spectra.[40] A new, recently introduced DSCT system uses an x-ray filter to remove the lowest energy photons from the high energy (eg, 140 kVp) spectrum. This yields greater separation of the low- and high-energy spectra and may reduce the overlap in attenuation values observed without the energy selective filter (**Fig. 6**).

A second approach to dual-energy CT imaging uses a single x-ray tube but alternates between two peak tube voltages during data acquisition and acquires two complete sets of projections during each gantry rotation. A third approach operates one x-ray tube at a single peak tube voltage to generate one distinct x-ray spectrum and uses layers of energy-sensitive detectors to capture both a low-energy and high-energy set of attenuated x-ray photons; lower energy radiation is absorbed by the top detector and higher energy radiation is absorbed by the bottom detector. Phantom work has demonstrated improved visualization of calcified coronary plaque[41] and coronary artery stent lumen[42] using dual energy.

Furthermore, from commercial realization is the use of photon-counting detection systems to acquire more than two spectrally distinct measurements. All of the approaches to dual-energy imaging described above are limited by the conventional CT detection systems used. Conventional systems integrate incoming x-ray photons without regard to spectral characteristics, inherently restricting energy resolution.[43] Photon-

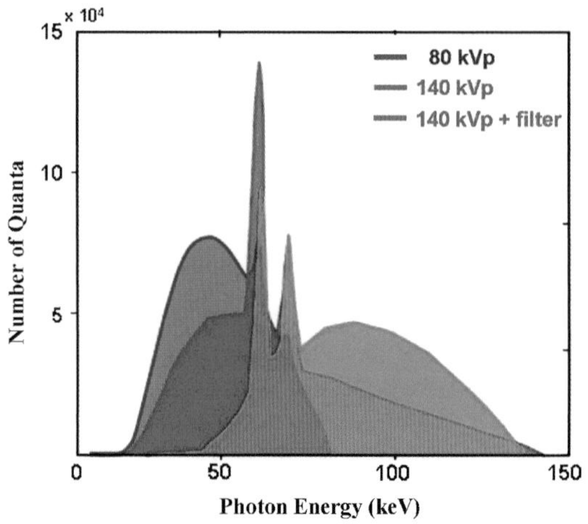


**Fig. 6.** X-ray spectra generated by applying a peak tube voltage of 80 kVp across an x-ray tube (*blue*), applying a peak tube voltage of 140 kVp across an x-ray tube (*red*), and applying a peak tube voltage of 140 kVp across an x-ray tube and filtering out the lowest energy photons (*green*). Filtering of the high-energy spectrum yields greater separation of the low- and high-energy spectra.

counting technology, however, permits discrimination of incoming photons; each x-ray event is assigned to one of multiple energy bins. Images are reconstructed using data from a single bin or a combination of bins. Preclinical results from multienergy CT have demonstrated the feasibility of using photon-counting detectors[44,45] and the potential for improvement in luminal depiction and plaque characterization.[45] However, challenges including limited gantry rotation speed because of slow count rates will delay clinical application, particularly to imaging of the heart.

## SUMMARY

Recent technical innovations in MDCT have resulted in lower radiation dose, improved temporal and spatial resolution, decreased scan time, and improved tissue differentiation.

The refinement of axial data acquisition for coronary imaging has enabled its use, rather than helical data acquisition, in coronary CT patients with low, stable heart rates, resulting in significant dose savings. Some systems permit anatomic-based tube-current modulation with ECG-triggered axial scanning, which can result in additional dose savings. For patients with contraindications to prospectively ECG-triggered axial imaging, the expanded flexibility of ECG-based tube-current modulation has resulted in lower doses with helical imaging.

Other advances aimed at lowering radiation dose for both axial and helical acquisitions include the use of adaptive prepatient *z*-collimators. Some CT systems use prepatient *z*-collimation to reduce x-ray exposure by preventing x-rays outside the planned scan length, but not contributing diagnostic information, from reaching the patient. In addition, implementation of iterative reconstruction algorithms is being explored for CT imaging in hopes of achieving a reduction in radiation dose without a loss in image quality.

Recent gains in temporal resolution have been achieved by some manufacturers by decreasing the gantry rotation time or increasing the number of x-ray sources from one to two. Recent improvements in spatial resolution have been less dramatic, although application of the flying focal spot technique in the *z*-direction has served to enhance *z*-resolution. Iterative reconstruction algorithms, however, offer the greatest potential for significant improvements in spatial resolution for cardiac CT.

Significant decreases in scan time have been accomplished with newer MDCT systems by increasing *z*-coverage per rotation through the design of detector arrays with increasing numbers of detector rows. A new approach to decreasing scan time is to significantly increase pitch through the simultaneous use of two x-ray sources. X-ray exposure is decreased by decreasing the amount of redundant data collected. Although extremely promising, this approach still requires clinical validation.

Attempts to gain spectral information from CT and improve tissue discrimination have resulted in the implementation of multiple approaches to dual-energy data acquisition. Early results demonstrate the added value of the additional attenuation information. The extraction of even more spectral information beyond that provided by dual-energy imaging may be possible through the use of photon-counting detectors.

## REFERENCES


1. Hounsfield GN. The E.M.I. scanner. Proc R Soc Lond B Biol Sci 1977;195:281–9.
2. Kalendar WA. Computed tomography: fundamentals, system technology, image quality, and applications. Germany: Publicis MCD Verlag; 2006.
3. Boyd DP, Lipton MJ. Cardiac computed tomography. Proc IEEE 1983;71:298–307.
4. Kalendar WA, Seissler W, Klotz E, et al. Spiral volumetric CT with single-breath-hold technique, continuous transport, and continuous scanner rotation. Radiology 1990;176:181–3.
5. Crawford CR, King KF. Computed tomography scanning with simultaneous patient translation. Med Phys 1990;17(6):967–82.
6. Carr JJ, Crouse JR, Goff DC, et al. Evaluation of subsecond gated helical CT for quantification of coronary artery calcium and comparison with electron beam CT. Am J Roentgenol 2000;174:915–21.
7. Becker CR, Jakobs TF, Aydemir S, et al. Helical and single-slice conventional CT versus electron beam CT for the quantification of coronary artery calcification. Am J Roentgenol 2000;174:543–7.
8. Klingenbeck-Regn K, Schaller S, Flohr T, et al. Subsecond multi-slice computed tomography: basics and applications. Eur J Radiol 1999;31:110–24.
9. Hu H, He HD, Foley WD, et al. Four multidectector-row helical CT: image quality and volume coverage speed. Radiology 2000;215:55–62.
10. Flohr T, Stierstorfer K, Bruder H, et al. New technical developments in multislice CT, part 1: Approaching isotropic resolution with sub-millimeter 16-slice scanning. Röfo: fortschritte auf dem Gebiet der Röntgenstrahlen und der bildgebenden Verfahren 2002;174(7):839–45.
11. Flohr T, Bruder H, Stierstorfer K, et al. New technical developments in multislice CT, part 2: Sub-millimeter 16-slice scanning and increased gantry rotation speed for cardiac imaging. Röfo: fortschritte auf dem Gebiet der Röntgenstrahlen und der bildgebenden Verfahren 2002;174(8):1022–7.
12. Flohr T, Stierstorfer K, Raupach R, et al. Performance evaluation of a 64-slice CT system with z-flying focal spot. Rofo 2004;176(12):1803–10.
13. Flohr TG, McCollough CH, Bruder H, et al. First performance evaluation of a dual-source (DSCT) system. Eur Radiol 2006;16:256–68.
14. Rybicki FJ, Otero HJ, Steigner ML, et al. Initial evaluation of coronary images from 320-detector row computed tomography. Int J Cardiovasc Imaging 2008;24:535–46.
15. Mettler FA, Huda W, Yoshizumi TT, et al. Effective doses in radiology and diagnostic nuclear medicine: a catalog. Radiology 2008;248:254–63.
16. Einstein AJ, Henzlova MJ, Rajagopalan S. Estimating risk of cancer associated with radiation exposure from 64-slice computed tomography coronary angiography. JAMA 2007;298(3):317–23.
17. Brenner DJ, Hall EJ. Computed tomography—an increasing source of radiation exposure. N Engl J Med 2007;357:2277–84.
18. Tzedakis A, Damilakis J, Perisinakis K, et al. The effect of z overscanning on patient effective dose from multi-detector helical computed tomography examinations. Med Phys 2005;32(6):1621–9.
19. Walker MJ, Olzsewki ME, Desai MY, et al. New radiation dose saving technologies for 256-slice cardiac computed tomography angiography. Int J Cardiovasc Imaging 2009;25:189–99.

20. Earls JP, Berman EL, Urban BA, et al. Prospectively gated transverse coronary CT angiography versus retrospectively gated helical technique: improved image quality and reduced radiation dose. Radiology 2008;246:742–53.
21. Stolzmann P, Leschka S, Scheffel H, et al. Dual-source CT in step-and shoot mode: noninvasive coronary angiography with low radiation dose. Radiology 2008;249:71–80.
22. Weigold WG, Olszewski ME, Walker MJ. Low-dose prospectively gated 256-slice coronary computed tomography angiography. Int J Cardiovasc Imaging 2009;25:217–30.
23. Kitagawa K, Lardo AC, George RT. Prospective ECG-gated 320 row detector computed tomography: implications for CT angiography and perfusion imaging. Int J Cardiovasc Imaging, in press.
24. Halliburton SS, Sola S, Kuzmiak SA, et al. Impact of dual source cardiac computed tomography on patient radiation dose in a clinical setting: comparison to single source imaging. J Cardiovasc Comput Tomogr 2008;2(6):392–400.
25. Hausleiter J, Meyer T, Hermann F, et al. Estimated radiation dose associated with cardiac CT angiography. JAMA 2009;301:500–7.
26. Mulkens TH, Bellinck P, Baeyaert M, et al. Use of an automatic exposure control mechanism for dose optimization in multi-detector row CT examinations: clinical evaluation. Radiology 2005;237:213–23.
27. McCollough CH, Primak AN, Saba O, et al. Dose performance of a 64-channel dual-source CT scanner. Radiology 2007;243:773–84.
28. Petersilka M, Bruder H, Krauss B, et al. Technical principles of dual source CT. Eur J Radiol 2008;68(3):362–8.
29. Thibault J, Sauer KD, Bouman CA, et al. A three-dimensional statistical approach to improved image quality for multislice helical CT. Med Phys 2007;34(11):4526–44.
30. Wang G, Yu H, De Man B. An outlook on x-ray CT research and development. Med Phys 2008;35(3):1051–64.
31. Flohr T, Raupach R, Bruder H, et al. How much can temporal resolution, spatial resolution and volume coverage be improved? J Cardiovasc Comput Tomogr 2009;3(3):143–52.
32. Engel KJ, Herrman C, Zeitler G. X-ray scattering in single- and dual-source CT. Med Phys 2007;35(1):318–32.
33. Mori S, Endo M, Komatsu S, et al. A combination-weighted Feldkamp-based reconstruction algorithm for cone-beam CT. Phys Med Biol 2006;51:3953–65.
34. Endo M, Mori S, Tsunoo T. Magnitude and effects of x-ray scatter in a 256-slice CT scanner. Med Phys 2006;33(9):3359–68.
35. Hameed TA, Teague SD, Vembar M, et al. Non-coronary CT chest angiography utilizing low radiation dose ECG gated imaging techniques of a 256 slice multidetector CT scanner. Int J Cardiovasc 2009;25:267–78.
36. McCullough EC. Photon attenuation in computed tomography. Med Phys 1975;2:307–20.
37. Alverez RE, Macovski A. Energy-selective reconstructions in x-ray computerized tomography. Phys Med Biol 1976;21:733–44.
38. Ruzsics B, Lee H, Zwerner PL, et al. Dual-energy CT of the heart for diagnosing coronary artery stenosis and myocardial ischemia-initial experience. Eur Radiol 2008;18(11):2414–24.
39. Schwarz F, Ruzsics B, Schoepf UJ, et al. Dual-energy CT of the heart—principles and protocols. Eur J Radiol 2008;68:423–33.
40. Barreto M, Schoenhagen P, Nair A. Potential of dual energy computed tomography to characterize atherosclerotic plaque: ex vivo assessment of human coronary arteries in comparison to histology. J Cardiovasc Comput Tomogr 2008;2(4):234–42.
41. Boll DT, Merkle EM, Paulson EK. Coronary stent patency: dual-energy multidetector CT assessment in a pilot study with anthropomorphic phantom. Radiology 2008;247(3):687–95.
42. Boll DT, Merkle EM, Paulson EK, et al. Calcified vascular plaque specimens: assessment with cardiac dual-energy multidetector CT in anthropomorphically moving heart phantom. Radiology 2008;249(1):119–26.
43. Alvarez RE, Seibert JA, Thompson SK. Comparison of dual energy detector system performance. Med Phys 2004;31(3):556–65.
44. Shikhaliev PM. Energy-resolved computed tomography: first experimental results. Phys Med Biol 2008;53:5595–613.
45. Feuerlein S, Roessl E, Proksa R. Multienergy photon-counting K-edge imaging: potential for improved luminal depiction in vascular imaging. Radiology 2008;249(3):1010–6.

# Radiation Dose and Safety in Cardiac Computed Tomography

Thomas C. Gerber, MD, PhD[a,b,*], Birgit Kantor, MD[c], Cynthia H. McCollough, PhD[d]

**KEYWORDS**

- Coronary artery disease • Coronary angiography
- Imaging • Computed tomography • Ionizing radiation
- Radiation risks • Patient outcomes
- Risk/benefit assessment

In recent years, reports on radiation exposure resulting from medical imaging have unfailingly attracted intense attention by the media, whose reporting typically emphasizes the risks of such exposure. It is certainly possible that the growing use of imaging procedures that rely on ionizing radiation may have significant effects on public health. However, the potential health risks of ionizing radiation at the levels used in medical imaging are rarely portrayed in a balanced fashion that would highlight the patterns of use of medical imaging, the uncertainties about the magnitude of risk of cancer, or the undeniable benefits of medical imaging in specific scenarios. The purpose of this article is to provide an understanding of (*i*) the strengths and shortcomings of epidemiologic evaluations of radiation exposure to the general population, (*ii*) the uncertainties related to radiation dosimetry and estimating the biologic risk (including carcinogenesis) resulting from exposure to ionizing radiation, and (*iii*) the measures that can be taken to maximize our opportunities to perform the right study in the right patient with a radiation dose that is as low as reasonably achievable. In keeping with the main theme of the current issue of *Cardiology Clinics*, this article focuses on cardiac computed tomography (CT) imaging in adults.

## RADIATION EXPOSURE OF THE GENERAL POPULATION

A preliminary report by the National Commission for Radiation Protection (NCRP) on the medical radiation exposures of the United States population in 2006[1] was mostly based on publicly available information from Medicare claims, Veterans Administration data, and information from the Agency for Health care Quality and Research. Among the nuclear medicine studies, which increased at a rate of 5% per year, cardiac imaging accounted for 57% of the procedures but 85% of the collective dose. CT imaging has received particular attention in recent reports of patient dose. In 2007, a review published in the *New England Journal of Medicine*[2] reported an increase of CT imaging procedures from about 3 million in 1980 to an estimated 62 million in 2006. The preliminary NCRP report from 2008 suggested an increase of CT imaging studies by greater than 10% per year. Among the CT studies performed in 2006, the estimated 800,000 coronary artery scoring and "gated cardiac studies" (representing coronary CT angiography) accounted for 1.3% of the procedures and 1.5% of the collective effective dose (E).

This article was supported in part by NIH Grant 1R01EB007986-02 ("Non-Invasive Localization of Vulnerable Plaques") (to B.K. and C.H.M.)

[a] Division of Cardiovascular Diseases, Mayo Clinic, 4500 San Pablo Road, Jacksonville, FL 32224, USA
[b] Department of Radiology, Mayo Clinic, 4500 San Pablo Road, Jacksonville, FL 32224, USA
[c] Division of Cardiovascular Diseases, Mayo Clinic, 200 First Street SW, Rochester, MN 55905, USA
[d] Department of Radiology, Mayo Clinic, 200 First Street SW, Rochester, MN 55905, USA
* Corresponding author.
*E-mail address:* gerber.thomas@mayo.edu (T.C. Gerber).

Cardiol Clin 27 (2009) 665–677
doi:10.1016/j.ccl.2009.06.006
0733-8651/09/$ – see front matter 

Taken together, the estimated 67 million CT and 19 million nuclear medicine studies performed in 2006 accounted for 22% of imaging procedures that used ionizing radiation but 75% of the collective E (expressed in person-Sieverts). As a result of the changes in use of imaging procedures that rely on ionizing radiation, the collective dose has increased by over 700% and the annual per-capita dose, by almost 600% (from 0.53 mSv to 3 mSv), compared with previous reports on the exposure of the United States population to ionizing radiation in general[3] and medical exposure in particular.[4]

The collective dose can be a useful index for quantifying doses in large populations but does not account for the fact that a large dose delivered to a small number of people is not the same as a small dose delivered to many people.[5] Some medical physicists consider the collective dose a highly speculative and uncertain measure of risk that should, at levels of less than 100 mSv above background radiation, not be used for the purpose of estimating population health risks.[5] The annualized per-capita doses were obtained by dividing the cumulative dose delivered to all patients by the size of the entire population, irrespective of age, occupation, location, or health status. This methodology does, for example, not account for the fact that 80% of the cumulative CT dose were delivered in the hospital setting, presumably in seriously ill in-patients.[6] In comparison, the annual dose to individuals not receiving medical exposures has not or only minimally changed since 1987. Furthermore, a disproportionately high number of CT imaging procedures is performed in the elderly. Put in perspective, it is quite conceivable that in the ill and the elderly, populations at increased risk of dying, medical imaging procedures that require ionizing radiation can allow management decisions that can improve quality of life or longevity, suggesting a favorable relationship between risks and benefits of radiation exposure in this patient group. Near the end of this article, this concept is discussed in the context of cardiac imaging.

## BIOLOGIC INJURY FROM RADIATION

Most of what is known about the biologic effects of ionizing radiation[7] is derived from ex vivo studies or from examining and following the survivors of the atomic bomb explosions in Hiroshima and Nagasaki. The effects of ionizing radiation depend on the dose and the rate at which the dose is delivered.

### *Markers of Radiation Injury*

The acute effects of ionizing radiation are mostly mediated through impaired cell renewal (at the stage of mitosis) and triggering of apoptosis (which may not occur until after several cycles of cell division). The radiation sensitivity of cells and tissues is related to the rate of cellular proliferation, number of future divisions, and degree of differentiation. Among the most sensitive tissues are the precursor cells of hematopoiesis and the intestinal epithelium. As a result, absolute counts and relative changes of circulating lymphocytes, and the time to onset of emesis, have emerged as useful semi-quantitative biologic markers of absorbed radiation doses exceeding 6 Gy.[8] Quantitative analysis of chromosomal aberrations of lymphocytes, mostly in the form of interchange between two separate chromosomes (dicentrics), in blood samples drawn greater than 24 hours after exposure, is the current reference standard for estimating the absorbed radiation dose in vivo.[9]

The dose-dependent effects of ionizing radiation fall into two categories. The severity of "deterministic" effects, which typically occur once tissue-specific thresholds are exceeded, varies with the dose. Examples for deterministic effects include the aforementioned influence on tissues with rapid turnover, but also hair loss and the development of skin erythema and cataracts. For "stochastic" effects, it is the probability, not severity, of occurrence that varies with dose, typically without an appreciable threshold and after a latency period that may last decades. The specific mechanisms that result in deterministic versus stochastic effects are not well known.

### *Risk of Carcinogenesis*

The stochastic radiation effect of greatest concern is carcinogenesis. The dose-response relationship between ionizing radiation at the levels used in medical imaging and the development of malignancies is controversial.[10] The data developed from survivors of atomic bomb explosions reflect uniform whole-body irradiation at high levels and energy in a specific Japanese population. It is not universally accepted that these data can be extrapolated to the highly nonuniform partial-body irradiation at much lower levels typical of medical imaging in other populations of various ethnicities.[5]

Several issues complicate the quantitative evaluation of carcinogenic risk related to ionizing radiation at effective doses less than 100 mSv (which reflects the definition of "low dose"). First, the effect appears to be small: neither in the Life Span Study of atomic bomb blast survivors[11] nor in retrospective epidemiologic analyses in radiation workers,[12] both studies with large sample sizes and long follow-up, was the risk of developing solid malignancies in the "low dose" range unequivocally different from no increased risk. It is important to realize that radiation-induced malignancies are indistinguishable from malignancies related to other carcinogens or biologic processes. Therefore, the small potential risk of carcinogenesis would be superimposed on, and difficult to differentiate from, the substantial intrinsic average lifetime risks in the United States of developing (41%) or dying from (21%) a malignancy.[13] This small potential would also vary greatly by sex, age, and health status of the individual. Finally, the general population is exposed to natural background radiation to geographically varying degrees that averages approximately 3.5 mSv per year. Given the random nature of the interaction of ionizing particles with critical cellular targets, it is conceivable that even the low levels of background radiation could contribute to the development of malignancies, which would be difficult to differentiate from the effects of a single exposure to medical radiation.

### *Relationship between low-dose radiation and risk of lethal malignancy*

Given the small potential effect and the large number of confounding factors, a study setting out to establish the relationship between low levels of radiation and the development of malignancies would require hundreds of thousands of study subjects and decades of follow-up. Given the facts that there is no definite evidence that suggests such a relationship exists but that a relationship cannot be ruled out, several professional societies or committees have endorsed the conservative assumption that the risk of malignancies at low doses of radiation can be extrapolated from the risk of malignancies at high levels of radiation, and that there is no dose of radiation that cannot potentially cause malignancies.[11,14] This concept is commonly referred to as the "linear no-threshold hypothesis" and is by no means universally accepted. A conceivable alternative "linear quadratic hypothesis" suggests that at low radiation doses the risk of malignancy is so low as to be unquantifiable in humans, but that the risk rises exponentially at higher doses. Yet another concept, termed "radiation hormesis," even implies that exposure to low levels of radiation can convey health and survival benefits.[15]

The public summary of the Biologic Effect of Ionizing Radiation VII report concedes that "statistical limitations make it difficult to evaluate cancer risk in humans" at doses of less than 100 mSv but overall the report endorses the linear no-threshold hypothesis.[11] The report quotes a 5 in 100 age- and gender-average lifetime risk of dying from a malignancy attributable to radiation exposure among individuals of the general population who received an effective dose of 1 Sv. This risk would translate into 1 in 2,000 patients (0.05%) who have received the 10-mSv dose that is typical of a coronary CT angiogram (CTA) acquired using a retrospective gating protocol.

A recent study modeled age- and gender-specific whole body and organ lifetime attributable risks (LAR) of cancer associated the radiation exposure from a 64-slice coronary CTA.[16] The computations were based on scanning protocols that used retrospective gating and generic Monte Carlo modeling of organ doses. The LARs were based on the linear no-threshold hypothesis. As expected, the risk varied by gender, age, and scanning protocol (**Table 1**), and ranged from 0.7% for 20-year-old women to 0.044% for 80-year-old men if no dose-sparing algorithm was used. The risks were 35% lower if dose-sparing algorithms were used. At all ages, lung and breast cancer combined accounted for 80% to 85% of the LAR in women.

## PARAMETERS TO QUANTIFY RADIATION DOSE

The objective of the design of scanner settings and scanning protocols is to obtain images of diagnostic quality. Image noise and motion artifacts are two key determinants of image quality in cardiac CT. The technical specifications that affect the temporal resolution of CT images and, hence, the probability of cardiac and coronary motion artifacts, are addressed in S. Halliburton's article "Recent technologic advances in multi-detector row cardiac CT" in this issue of *Cardiology Clinics* and have limited effect on patient dose. Conversely, the scanner settings that affect image noise also greatly affect X-ray tube output and patient dose.

### *Relationship of Scanner Settings, Tube Output, and Image Quality*

Image noise is inversely proportional to the number of photons received by the detector array. The product of tube current multiplied by exposure time (expressed in units of milliAmpere seconds), the tube voltage (expressed in units of peak kiloVolt, kVp), the reconstructed slice width, and the degree of photon attenuation are the main determinants of the number of photons received by the detector array.[17] The milliAmpere seconds mainly increases photon flux, and the peak kVp kiloVolt, photon energy. Photon attenuation increases with

**Table 1**
**Estimated risk of cancer incidence attributable to a single coronary computed tomographic angiogram based on the linear no-threshold hypothesis**

| Gender | Age (Years) | Risk |
|---|---|---|
| Female | 20 | 0.7% (1 in 143) |
| Female | 40 | 0.35% (1 in 286) |
| Female | 60 | 0.22% (1 in 546) |
| Female | 80 | 0.075% (1 in 1333) |
| Male | 20 | 0.15% (1 in 667) |
| Male | 40 | 0.099% (1 in 1010) |
| Male | 60 | 0.081% (1 in 1235) |
| Male | 80 | 0.044% (1 in 2273) |

Data reflect no dose-sparing algorithm used. Effective dose for women, 21 mSv; effective dose for men, 15 mSv. Risks were 35% lower if electrocardiographically tube-current modulation was used as a dose-sparing scanning protocol. (*Data from* Einstein AJ, Henzlova MJ, Rajagopalan S. Estimating risk of cancer associated with radiation exposure from 64-slice computed tomography coronary angiography. JAMA 2007;298:317.)

increases in body thickness. Therefore, adaptation of default scanner settings to a patient's body size can be needed to avoid excessive image noise that could interfere with confident image interpretation. For example, for every 4 cm to 5 cm of additional tissue to be traversed by photons, the scanner output must be doubled for the level of image noise to remain constant.

Because patient dose is related to photon flux and energy, heavier patients may receive a higher dose of radiation (typically achieved by increasing milliAmpere seconds) to obtain images of diagnostic quality. Therefore, comparisons of doses between different CT scanning protocols are only meaningful at comparable levels of image noise. Because most of the additional dose is absorbed by the external fatty tissue, organ doses do not increase linearly with milliAmpere seconds.[18] In this context, it is interesting to note that body weight is not an ideal predictor of tube output requirements in cardiac CT because increases in weight often reflect increased abdominal, not necessarily thoracic, thickness.[19]

## Measurable Parameters in Radiation Dosimetry

The radiation output of CT scanners can be assessed in several ways. Parameters of radiation output that can be measured or calculated from measured values with standardized procedures lend themselves for the determination of diagnostic reference levels. Diagnostic reference levels are useful benchmarks for quality assurance efforts to identify practices that deliver, for specific radiologic examinations, doses far above their peers. Diagnostic reference levels are typically set at the seventy-fifth to eightieth percentile of clinical-dose surveys.[20,21] Consistently exceeding diagnostic reference levels suggests the need for local review and practice adaptation. The use of diagnostic reference levels for benchmarking can reduce the median dose and dose variability, as assessed in periodic surveys.[22,23]

### *Computed tomographic dose index*

Most of the parameters used to measure radiation output were originally developed for imaging protocols that acquired single, parallel, transaxial slices, and can be applied to modern multidetector CT technology only with modifications. The computed tomography dose index (CTDI), a basic radiation-dose parameter in CT, is defined as the integral under the radiation-dose profile of a single rotation scan at a fixed table position divided by the nominal width of the radiation beam (**Fig. 1**).[24] The normalization to the nominal width of the radiation profile builds a "dose efficiency" factor into the value. Several variants of the CTDI exist that have been detailed elsewhere in terms relevant to clinicians.[17,25] In short, the $CTDI_{100}$ represents a specific mode of measuring radiation exposure (in units of Coulomb/kilogram) with an ionization chamber of 100-mm length. The weighted CTDI ($CTDI_w$) is a calculated measure of the average absorbed dose in the scan plane (*x*- and *y*-axes) that is obtained from several $CTDI_{100}$ measurements.

The volume CTDI ($CTDI_{vol}$; in units of milliGray, mGy) represents the average radiation within a specific volume and is now the preferred standardized measure of radiation output in CT dosimetry.[17,25,26] The $CTDI_{vol}$ is convenient because it is derived from the easily measured $CTDI_{100}$, and it is useful for comparisons between different imaging protocols because it incorporates protocol-specific information on the spatial separation or overlap between successive scans. In helical CT, this spatial relationship between successive scans is dependent on the advance of the patient table during each gantry rotation (pitch). As a conceptual disadvantage, the $CTDI_{vol}$ does not reflect the total number of scans that make up a CT examination.

### *Dose-length product*

The dose-length product (DLP) best represents the integrated radiation output during a specific complete CT examination.[17,25,26] The DLP (in units of mGy $\times$ cm) is defined as the $CTDI_{vol}$ multiplied

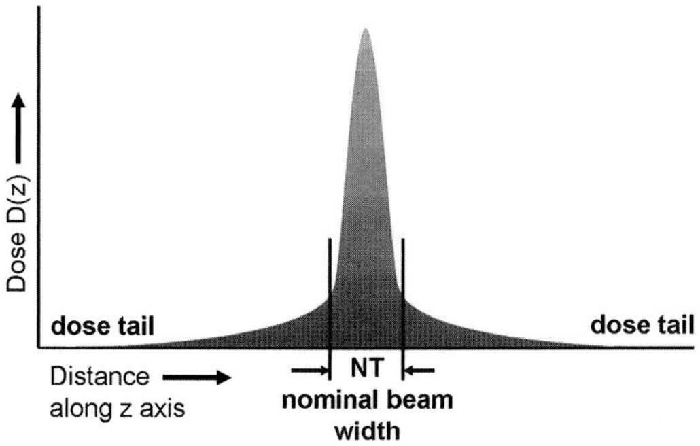


**Fig. 1.** Distribution of radiation dose of a single axial CT scan along the *z*-axis, perpendicular to the scan plane. The tails on either side of the dose profile are the result of X-ray beam divergence and internal radiation scatter. The CTDI is defined as the integral under the area under the curve normalized to the nominal beam width (NT). (*From* Bauhs JA, Vrieze TJ, Primak AN, et al. CT dosimetry: comparison of measurement techniques and devices. Radiographics 2008;28:246; with permission.)

by the scan length. The typical scan length for a coronary CTA is 12 cm. Because the numeric value of the DLP can vary with patient anatomy, the $CTDI_{vol}$ is more useful than the DLP for designing and comparing CT scanning protocols.

## *Estimates of Radiation Dose*

The effective dose (in units of milliSievert) is a generic, calculated approximation of the biologic detriment (ie, the stochastic risk) of a nonhomogeneous body irradiation such as that which occurs during medical imaging of specific body regions. E represents the mean absorbed whole-body dose that would result in the same total radiation detriment as the nonuniform partial-body irradiation in question. There is no measurable physical gold standard that represents E.[10,17,25,26]

E is estimated in three steps.[27] First, the so-called "Monte Carlo" simulation is used to estimate the radiation doses (in units of milliGray) received by individual organs. Monte Carlo simulation models the scattering of photons and the resulting absorption of radiation energy in standardized mathematical models of the human body: for example, that of a man with a weight of 70 kg. The amount of ionization, and hence the probability of a relevant biologic effect, along the track of an ionizing particle passing through the body varies between low (eg, X-rays) and high (eg, alpha particles) linear energy-transfer sources. Therefore, in a second step in the estimation of E, the relative biologic effectiveness of different types of ionizing radiation is represented by a radiation weighting factor. For X-rays, the radiation weighting factor is 1. As discussed in the section "Biologic injury from radiation" above, the radiation sensitivity of different tissues varies considerably. Therefore, the third step in the estimation of E applies tissue-specific weighting factors that represent the radiation sensitivity of each organ or tissue. These tissue-specific weighting factors determine how much the individual organ doses contribute when E is calculated as the sum of the products obtained by multiplying organ doses with radiation and tissue-specific weighting factors.

The tissue-specific weighting factors are determined from population averages in the survivors of atomic bomb explosions. Because of the evolving knowledge of the biology and epidemiology of radiation injuries, several sets of tissue weighting factors exist. For example, the International Commission for Radiation Protection (ICRP) published slightly differing sets in 1977,[28] 1991,[29] and 2007.[30] In addition, methodologic differences in the calculation of E exist between the three ICRP recommendations. These differences pertain, for example, to the incorporation of the so-called "remainder tissues" or tissues for which no organ coefficients exist, and to the best method of averaging dose over an organ. As a result, the numerical value of E can vary because of methodologic differences alone, even if the actual radiation exposure is identical. **Table 2** gives an example of how the E of a coronary CT angiogram obtained with a typical single-source 64-slice scanning protocol ($CTDI_{vol,}$ 59.9 mGy) might vary based on the various ICRP recommendations.

The European Working Group for Guidelines on Quality Criteria in CT has suggested a simplified method for the estimation of E. This estimate is obtained by multiplying the DLP with a conversion coefficient that varies dependent on which body region is scanned. The conversion coefficient for the thorax,[31] which is relevant for cardiac CT, was recently revised from 0.017 mSv to 0.014 $mSv \times mGy^{-1} \times cm^{-1}$.

It is important to recognize that E is not an exact indicator of patient-specific absolute biologic risk because is does not take into account variations of human anatomy (eg, body weight at the upper and lower end of the spectrum) and because uncertainties about the radiation risk of human tissues remain.[10] Because of the generic modeling and the many uncertainties relating to organ dose and organ risks, E should be reported as ranges rather than single numerical values with several significant figures.[32] To obtain risk estimates that apply to individual patients, exact organ doses and organ-specific risk estimates related to age and gender are needed. This type of modeling is extraordinarily complex. Nonetheless, E is useful

**Table 2**
**Differences in effective dose estimates based on the recommendations in three publications from the ICRP**

| ICRP Publication | 26 | 60 | 103 |
|---|---|---|---|
| Year | 1977 | 1990 | 2007 |
| Breast weighting coefficient | 0.15 | 0.05 | 0.12 |
| E (mSv) | 25 | 17 | 22 |
| Percent difference[a] | 151% | 100% | 134% |

Data are for a single-source 64 detector-row multislice coronary CT angiogram (volume CTDI, 60 mGy). The differences in E are related to changing values of the tissue-weighting coefficient of the breast, the handling of remainder tissues, and dose averaging.

[a] The recommendations in ICRP publication 60, still widely used, were used as a reference to calculate relative differences in E between the three recommendations.

for comparisons of the biologic effect of different imaging protocols, different types of radiologic examinations, or even between imaging modalities that use different types of ionizing radiation. E can also help patients put the risk of a proposed radiologic examination in perspective by comparison with the E received from natural background radiation (average, 3 mSv per year; range, 1 mSv–10 mSv). However, comparisons between E should keep the diagnostic objective in mind. Interpreting the E of a typical coronary CTA of 12 mSv as the equivalent of 600 chest X-rays or 1,200 panoramic dental X-rays may not be meaningful, because neither chest X-rays nor dental X-rays are necessarily helpful in establishing or ruling out coronary artery disease as the cause of chest pain in a symptomatic patient.

## TECHNIQUES TO REDUCE RADIATION DOSE

Given the oft-cited increase of cumulative and per-capita dose related to medical imaging in recent years, it is easily overlooked that, as a result of improvements in scanner technology and dose efficiency, the mean radiation dose per type of examination in general has decreased by a factor of 2 to 3 over the past two decades.[33] Recently developed scanning protocols allow tremendous reduction of radiation dose in cardiovascular imaging on state-of-the-art multidetector CT scanners.

Certainly, considering on a per-patient basis whether the findings of a cardiac CT are likely to affect management meaningfully, and foregoing the study if it will not, must stand at the top of the hierarchy of dose-saving strategies. However, in this context it is equally important that the treating health care provider considers the risks of not performing a cardiac CT—that is, the risk of missing an important diagnosis—if the examination is not performed because of concerns about radiation dose.[10] As a second basic measure, to be addressed by the health care provider performing the imaging study, the scan length should be limited to include only the structures of interest, without routinely adding a "safety margin" above and below the heart.

Traditionally, cardiac-scanning protocols with multidetector CT use continuous radiation output from the X-ray tube throughout the cardiac cycle.[34] However, the images, typically reconstructed retrospectively within a short time window during the diastolic period of the cardiac cycle, represent only a small fraction of the radiation dose received. Given the relationships between X-ray tube settings and radiation dose detailed above, most dose-reduction strategies in cardiac CT rely on reduction of tube voltage or tube current or both for a part or for all of the cardiac cycle. Some techniques of dose reduction that can be used for CT examinations of other body parts (eg, automatic exposure control) are not available for, or not effective in, cardiac CT.[18]

### *Tube-current Modulation*

As discussed above in the section on the relationship between scanner settings and image quality, photon attenuation is dependent upon the thickness and density of the body tissue to be traversed. The ovoid shape of the thorax, and the different densities along the length of the human body, lend themselves to tube-current modulation based on human anatomy. Angular (*x,y*) tube-current modulation[26] exploits the fact that the attenuation of the X-ray beam is higher when it traverses the body laterally than when it traverses the body from anterior or posterior locations. Therefore, during individual rotations of the gantry, the nominal tube current set by the operator is used only while scanning laterally, and can be reduced by the scanner while scanning occurs in anteroposterior or posteroanterior direction.

Similarly, attenuation of X-rays is higher near the bony structures of shoulder or hip regions than over the lungs or abdomen, and tube current can be adjusted by longitudinal (*z*) modulation[26] accordingly throughout the table advance through the gantry. However, angular and longitudinal tube-current modulation are currently not fully compatible with the approach of electrocardiographically controlled tube current modulation (ECTCM) discussed in the following section.

### *Electrocardiographically controlled tube-current modulation*

ECTCM is a dose-sparing algorithm specific to cardiovascular CT. If high-quality reconstruction of the projection data into planar images is needed for only one time point of the cardiac cycle (such as for coronary CTA), the tube current can be reduced during the parts of the cardiac cycle that are unlikely to be used for reconstruction. With ECTCM, nominal tube current is maintained during a time window of fixed length that can be determined by the operator, but typically is set in late diastole, and the tube current is reduced to approximately 20% during the remainder of the cardiac cycle (**Fig. 2**).[18,19] During the scan, the desired time window is identified prospectively based on the ECG. The length of the window of nominal tube current varies between different makes of scanners, and is programmable in some scanners. The effectiveness of ECTCM depends on the length of the window of nominal tube current, the level to which tube current is lowered for the remainder of the cardiac cycle, and the heart rate. ECTCM is more effective at low heart rates. In various studies, ECTCM has lowered the effective dose by between approximately 28% and 45%.[35–38]

As a disadvantage, images reconstructed from projection data acquired during periods of reduced tube current will be noisy, and pathologic anatomic or functional findings that depend on incorporating these images into overall assessment of the examination may not be readily recognized. The low quality of images reconstructed during periods of low tube current may also be disadvantageous in patients with higher heart rates, where optimal image quality with the least degree of motion artifact is often found during systole.[39] In addition, ECTCM is not reliable in patients with arrhythmia or pronounced extrasystole because the ECTCM algorithm may not identify the systolic and diastolic phase of the cardiac cycle correctly in this situation and may accidentally lower the tube current during the phase of the cardiac cycle that is desirable as a reconstruction window.

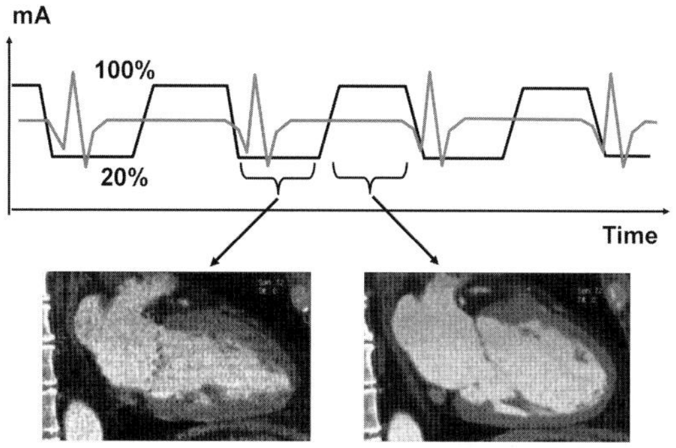


**Fig. 2.** Principle of ECG-controlled tube-current modulation. The tube current is a nominal value (100%) for a prospectively selected interval during diastole when images will likely be reconstructed (*right*). During the remainder of the cardiac cycle, tube current is reduced to 20%, which results in high image noise in images reconstructed during systole (*left*), but overall radiation dose to the patient is reduced. (*From* Paul JF, Abada HT. Strategies for reduction of radiation dose in cardiac multislice CT. Eur Radiol 2007;17:2030; with permission.)

## *Sequential Scanning*

Sequential scanning, sometimes referred to as "step-and-shoot," is a technique new to multidetector CT scanning.[18,40] In this approach, the X-ray tube is "on," prospectively triggered by the ECG, during only the part of the cardiac cycle to be used for image reconstruction, typically in late diastole. Given the fact that radiation is produced during only a part of the cardiac cycle, the dose reduction that can be achieved by this technique is very substantial, on the order of 77% to 87%. As a disadvantage, no projection data are acquired or available for image reconstructions during other parts of the cardiac cycle. Therefore, this approach is not useful for CT examinations meant to assess functional aspects of the heart throughout the cardiac cycle. To maximize the probability of obtaining images of diagnostic quality, CT centers experienced in coronary CTA with use of sequential scanning recommend rigorous patient selection. Selection criteria include a heart rate of no more then 65 to 75 beats per minute and a heart rate variability of less than 10 beats per minute.[41]

## *Individual Adaptation of Tube Voltage and Current*

Although "underexposure" of CT images is readily apparent in the form of image noise, "overexposure" in the form of areas that are too bright or too dark does not occur because of the normalization of CT data relative to water.[18] Therefore, opportunities to reduce radiation dose by decreasing tube voltage or tube current, which will decrease radiation output, are currently not always realized. In theory, radiation dose is linearly related to tube current, and exponentially related to the square of the difference between tube voltage settings. Therefore, reducing tube voltage is a more effective means of reducing radiation dose. As an added benefit, the increased attenuation by iodine of photons at lower photon energy (as it occurs with reduction of tube voltage) increases the contrast between the contrast-enhanced coronary artery lumen and the surrounding tissue. This advantage must be weighed against the increased image noise that results from higher attenuation of low-energy photons by the patient's body.

Several investigators have suggested reducing tube voltage from the standard 120 kVp to 100 kVp in patients with a body weight up to 75 kg or 85 kg. In one previous study, the combined use of tube voltage reduction and ECTCM resulted in a reduction of the E received from coronary CTA performed with single-source 64-slice MDCT by 64%, without appreciable reduction of subjectively perceived image quality.[36]

### *Barriers to the Consistent Use of Dose-saving Imaging Strategies*

Among the strategies for radiation dose reduction, ECTCM was used in 73% of patients, sequential scanning (prospective triggering) in 6%, and reduction of tube voltage from typically 120 kVp to 100 kVp in 5% of examinations in a recent international multicenter survey of radiation dose in cardiac CT.[42] When interpreting this pattern of use of dose-reduction strategies, it should be noted that at the time the survey was conducted in 2007 sequential scanning was not widely available. In addition, even at the time of this writing, the evidence base supporting the use of sequential scanning or reduced tube voltage is not as convincing as it is for ECTCM. Because of concerns that the use of these newer techniques might interfere with image quality to an extent that would reduce in a sizable number of examinations, the confidence with which they can be interpreted may have contributed to the limited use of sequential scanning and tube voltage reduction. It should also be clearly understood that certain dose-saving strategies cannot be used in certain patients or for examinations performed for functional imaging. Examples include patients with a very fast or irregular heart rate, obese patients, or CT examinations performed to assess left ventricular or valvular function. Studies are currently underway that examine the effect of sequential scanning or tube voltage reduction not only on image quality but also on diagnostic accuracy of coronary CTA.

## CURRENT RADIATION DOSE VALUES

Reliable data on dose estimates for various cardiac imaging procedures are not easily obtained. This is mainly because of (*i*) the uncertainties in the biologic risk of ionizing radiation, (*ii*) the generic and imprecise nature of radiation dose estimation that results in part from these uncertainties, and (*iii*) the fact that the current requirements for radiation dose reporting in individual institutions by the U.S. Food and Drug Administration, American College of Radiology accreditation surveys, and the National Regulatory Commission do not translate into easily available public information.

A catalog of values and ranges of E in radiology and diagnostic nuclear medicine was compiled recently from a review of the literature between 1980 and 2007.[43] A Science Advisory from the American Heart Association on ionizing radiation in cardiac imaging published in February 2009 modified and added to this information. **Table 3** shows representative values and ranges of effective dose estimates from the literature for various radiologic imaging studies.

The results of a first international survey of radiation dose in 1,965 cardiac CTA studies at 50 study sites were recently published.[42] As a particular strength, this study reported not only effective dose estimates but also $CTDI_{vol}$ and DLP as measurable dosimetry parameters. Therefore, this article reports the first and only set of diagnostic reference levels for cardiac CT available to date. Based on their findings, the authors suggested a $CTDI_{vol}$ of 70 mGy and a DLP of 1,200 mGy $\times$ cm as reference levels for coronary CTA for patients of average size.

An approximately sixfold variability of DLP (range, 331 mGy–2,146 mGy $\times$ cm) between study sites was observed. There were no significant differences of DLP by geographic location (**Fig. 3**). Multivariate regression analysis suggested the main determinants of the variability of radiation dose between sites were the user preferences for image noise, reconstruction algorithms kernel-determining in-pane sharpness, slice width (*z*-axis resolution), tube voltage (iodine contrast), and increased upper and lower limits of the scan range as a "safety zone," as well as patient size. The predictors for DLP in multivariate regression analysis are detailed in **Table 4**.

## SUMMARY AND PRACTICAL IMPLICATIONS

The risk of causing a malignancy at the radiation-dose levels used in cardiac imaging is hypothetical, not proven, and estimates of radiation dose

**Table 3**
**Representative values and ranges of effective dose estimates reported in the literature for selected radiologic studies**

| Examination | Representative Effective Dose Value (mSv) | Range of Reported Effective Dose Values (mSv) | Administered Activity (MBq) |
|---|---|---|---|
| Chest X-ray PA and lateral | 0.1 | 0.05–0.24 | NA |
| CT chest | 7 | 4–18 | NA |
| CT abdominal | 8 | 4–25 | NA |
| CT pelvis | 6 | 3–10 | NA |
| Coronary calcium CT[a] | 3 | 1–12 | NA |
| Coronary CTA | 16 | 5–32 | NA |
| 64-Slice coronary CTA | — | — | — |
| Without tube-current modulation | 15 | 12–18 | NA |
| With tube-current modulation[21] | 9 | 8–18 | NA |
| Dual-source coronary CTA | — | — | — |
| With tube current modulation | 13 | 6–17 | NA |
| Prospectively triggered coronary CTA[22] | 3 | 2–4 | NA |
| Diagnostic invasive coronary angiogram | 7 | 2–16 | NA |
| Percutaneous coronary intervention or radiofrequency ablation | 15 | 7–57 | NA |
| Myocardial perfusion study | — | — | — |
| Sestamibi (1-day) stress/rest | 9 | — | 1100 |
| Thallium stress/rest | 41 | — | 185 |
| F-18 FDG | 14 | — | 740 |
| Rubidium-82 | 5 | — | 1480 |

Includes data published between 1980 and 2007. Dose data may not reflect newest scanners and protocols.

64-Slice multidetector-row CT and dual-source CT studies published since 2005 only; data include a survey of the literature by Gerber and colleagues.[10]

*Abbreviations:* FDG, Fluorodeoxyglucose; NA, Not applicable; PA, Posteroanterior.

[a] Data combine prospectively triggered and retrospectively gated protocols. The representative effective dose is approximately 1 mSv for prospectively triggered coronary calcium CT scans and 3 mSv for retrospectively gated scans.

*Data from* Mettler F, Jr., Huda W, Yoshizumi T, Mahesh M. A catalog of effective doses in radiology and nuclear medicine. Radiology 2008;248:254 *and* Gerber TC, Carr JJ, Arai AE, et al. Ionizing radiation in cardiac imaging: a science advisory from the American Heart Association Committee on Cardiac Imaging of the Council on Clinical Cardiology and Committee on Cardiovascular Imaging and Intervention of the Council on Cardiovascular Radiology and Intervention. Circulation 2009;119:1056.

have a wide margin of error. However, in the absence of certainty, the consensus opinions of influential expert panels advocate adopting a conservative estimate of radiation risks. The median effective dose estimate for coronary CTA in a recent international survey of radiation doses in cardiac CTA (12 mSv) is in the same range as that of a 1-day myocardial scintigraphy stress test using Tc-99m sestamibi (9 mSv).[10] Information in that survey reflected the status quo of CT scanner technology in 2007. In the meantime, sophisticated CT imaging protocols that use prospective triggering of radiation dose output have become widely available, and can reduce the effective dose estimates to a fraction (2 mSv–4 mSv) of that of retrospectively gated protocols.

Radiation protection for patients involves justification, optimization, and limitation of exposure. How can we use all this complex information in making medical decisions that have the best

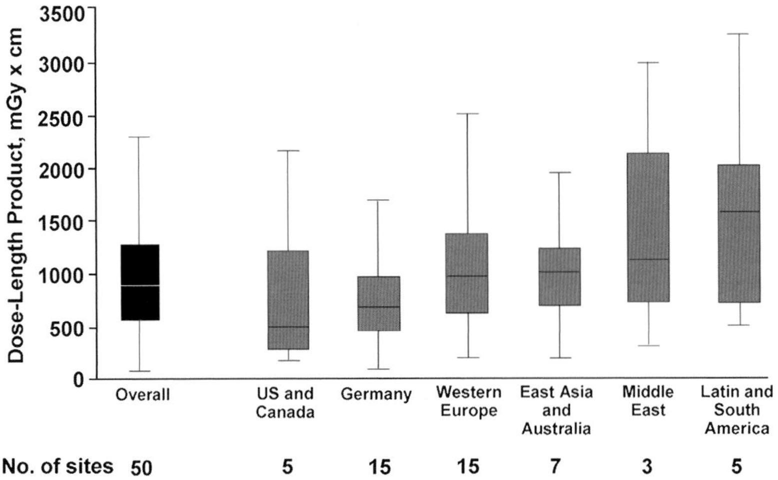


**Fig. 3.** Box-and-whiskers plot of dose-length product overall and by geographic location of study sites. Middle horizontal line, median; upper and lower edges of boxes, twenty-fifth and seventy-fifth percentiles of the interquartile range (IQR), respectively; lower whiskers, twenty-fifth percentile minus 1.5 times IQR; upper whiskers, seventy-fifth percentile plus 1.5 times IQR. (*From* Hausleiter J, Meyer T, Hermann F, et al. Estimated radiation dose associated with cardiac CT angiography. JAMA 2009;301:503; with permission.)

interest of the patient at heart? A recent Science Advisory from the American Heart Association[10] put forth a basic conceptual framework. Ultimately, the goal is to choose the right test for the right patient.

Coronary CTA is a highly accurate technique for defining the presence of coronary artery disease. Given the potential consequences of failing to identify coronary artery disease in symptomatic patients, one could consider the small hypothetical risk justified. In addition, the patient cohort of symptomatic patients with intermediate probability of coronary artery disease is predominantly older than 50 years of age, and many of these patients may well die from other (including cardiac) causes before such a malignancy can become clinically apparent. Conversely, coronary CTA may not be a proven or recommended screening tool for asymptomatic, low-risk patients, given the fact that, at this time, no data support the concept of using imaging evidence for "subclinical" atherosclerosis as a basis for management decisions. In the asymptomatic patient group, the small hypothetical risk may outweigh the unproven, potential benefit.

For now, cardiac CT should be ordered consistent with established appropriateness criteria and expert consensus.[44–46] Clearly, an individualized consideration of risks and benefits of cardiac CT in each patient is needed, and ideally risks and benefits should be discussed with the patient whenever practical. Can the clinical question at hand be addressed by means that do not use ionizing radiation? Has the patient perhaps recently at another institution undergone an imaging procedure that involved ionizing radiation that could help address the clinical question? Which among the appropriate imaging modalities will expose the patient to the least amount of radiation? These considerations should also include the risk of missing an important, potentially life-threatening diagnosis if imaging is not performed because of concerns about radiation. If a cardiac CT is deemed necessary, the available scanning options to reduce radiation dose that apply to the type of examination and the individual patient should be used unless justified reasons exist not to do so. Foregoing one-size-fits-all approaches to cardiac CT in favor of individualizing scanning protocols represents an all-important opportunity to keep patient dose as low as reasonably achievable.

It is up to the cardiac imaging community to develop the information needed to make rational determinations of the potential risk and benefits in individual patients. Emphasizing the importance and use of measurable X-ray tube output metrics in cardiac CT and routinely including such information in the imaging record to facilitate the determination of diagnostic reference levels and trends will help us understand to what levels of radiation dose patients are exposed with each permutation of scanner technology. In the clinical realm, studies of the value of detecting subclinical atherosclerosis in the form of noncalcified plaque for improving longevity are difficult to conceive and conduct, but are pivotal if the use of cardiac CT in asymptomatic patients with risk factors is

**Table 4**
**Predictors for dose-length product in multivariate linear regression analysis**

| Predictors | Effects (%) (95% CI) | *P* |
|---|---|---|
| Patient weight, 10-kg increase | 5 (4 to 6) | <0.001 |
| Indication, noncoronary versus coronary | −1 (−5 to 4) | 0.31 |
| Heart rhythm, nonsinus versus sinus | 10 (2 to 19) | 0.01 |
| Heart rate, 10-bpm increase | 1 (−1 to 1) | 0.98 |
| Scan length, 1-cm increase | 5 (4 to 6) | <0.001 |
| Automated exposure control | 0 (−3 to 3) | 0.97 |
| ECTCM[b] | −25 (−23 to −28) | <0.001 |
| Tube voltage 100 kV versus ≥120 kV or greater | −46 (−42 to −51) | <0.001 |
| Sequential versus spiral scanning | −78 (−77 to −79) | <0.001 |
| Site experience in CCTA, 12-mo increase | −1 (−1 to 0) | 0.03 |
| Performed CCTAs/mo, 10-CCTA increase | 0 (0 to 1) | 0.03 |
| 64-slice CT system versus Siemens single-source 64[c] | — | — |
| GE 64 | 97 (88 to 106) | <0.001 |
| Philips 64 | 11 (5 to 19) | <0.001 |
| Siemens dual-source 64 | 23 (17 to 30) | <0.001 |
| Toshiba 64 | 59 (47 to 71) | <0.001 |

*Abbreviations:* BPM, Beats per minute; CCTA, Cardiac CTA; CI, Confidence interval; CT, Computed tomography.
[a] Predictors for radiation dose are presented as % change in DLP (mGy × cm).
[b] Electrocardiographically controlled tube-current modulation.
[c] The Siemens single-source 64-slice CT system with the lowest median DLP in this study was used as a reference. The association with DLP is shown for the remaining four 64-slice systems within the linear regression analysis.
*Data from* Hausleiter J, Meyer T, Hermann F, et al. Estimated radiation dose associated with cardiac CT angiography. JAMA 2009;301(5):500–7.

to be justified. These efforts are needed to understand in which circumstances cardiac CT conveys benefit to patients by facilitating management decisions that will help them live better and longer.

## REFERENCES

1. Mettler F Jr, Thomadsen B, Bhargavan M, et al. Medical radiation exposure in the U.S. 2006 preliminary results. Health Phys 2008;95(5):502–7.
2. Brenner DJ, Hall EJ. Computed tomography—an increasing source of radiation exposure. N Engl J Med 2007;357(22):2277–84.
3. National Council on Radiation Protection and Measurements. Ionizing radiation exposure of the population of the United States: recommendations of the National Council on Radiation Protection and Measurements. Bethesda (MD): National Council on Radiation Protection and Measurements (NCRP); 1987. p. 93.
4. National Council on Radiation Protection and Measurements. Exposure of the U.S. Population from Diagnostic Medical Radiation: recommendation of the National Council on Radiation Protection and Measurements. Bethesda (MD): National Council on Radiation Protection and Measurements (NCRP); 1989. p. 100.
5. Health Physics Society. Radiation risk in perspective.http://hps.org/documents/risk_ps010-1.pdf. Accessed March 12, 2009.
6. National Council on Radiation Protection and Measurements. Ionizing radiation exposure of the population of the United States (prepublication copy). Bethesda, (MD): National Council on Radiation Protection and Measurements (NCRP); 2009. p. 160.
7. Hall EJ, Giaccia AJ. Radiation biology for the radiologist. Philadelphia: Lippincott, Williams and Wilkins; 2006.
8. Goans RE. Clinical care of the radiation accident patient: patient presentation, assessment and initial diagnosis. In: Ricks RC, Berger ME, O'Hare FM, editors. The medical basis for radiation accident preparedness: the clinical care of victims. Boca Raton (FL): Parthenon Publishing Group; 2002. p. 11–22.
9. Lloyd DC, Edwards AA, Moquet JE, et al. The role of cytogenetics in early triage of radiation casualties. Appl Radiat Isot 2000;52(5):1107–12.
10. Gerber TC, Carr JJ, Arai AE, et al. Ionizing radiation in cardiac imaging: a science advisory from the

American Heart Association Committee on cardiac imaging of the council on clinical cardiology and committee on cardiovascular imaging and intervention of the council on cardiovascular radiology and intervention. Circulation 2009;119(7):1056–65.
11. Committee to Assess Health Risks from Exposure to Low Levels of Ionizing Radiation, Board on Radiation Effects, Research Division on Earth and Life Studies, National Research Council of the National Academies. Health risks from exposure to low levels of ionizing radiation: BEIR VII-Phase 2. Washington, DC: National Academies Press; 2006.
12. Cardis E, Vrijheid M, Blettner M, et al. The 15-Country Collaborative Study of Cancer Risk among Radiation Workers in the Nuclear Industry: estimates of radiation-related cancer risks. Radiat Res 2007; 167:396–416.
13. Ries LAG, Melbert DK, Krapcho M, et al. Lifetime risk (percent) of being diagnosed with cancer and lifetime risk (percent) of dying from cancer, by site and race/ethnicity. SEER Cancer Statistic Review, 1975–2004; based on November 2006 SEER data submission, posted to the SEER Web site, 2007. Tables I–14 and I–17. Available at: http://seer.cancer.gov/csr/1975_2005/results_merged/topic_lifetime_risk.pdf. Accessed March 13, 2009.
14. National Council on Radiation Protection and Measurements. Risk estimates for radiation protection. Bethesda, (MD): National Council on Radiation Protection and Measurements (NCRP); 1993. p. 115.
15. Wikipedia - the free encyclopedia. Radiation hormesis. Available at: http://en.wikipedia.org/wiki/Radiation_hormesis. Accessed March 12, 2009.
16. Einstein AJ, Henzlova MJ, Rajagopalan S. Estimating risk of cancer associated with radiation exposure from 64-slice computed tomography coronary angiography. JAMA 2007;298(3):317–23.
17. Gerber TC, Kuzo RS, Morin RL. Techniques and parameters for estimating radiation exposure and dose in cardiac computed tomography. Int J Cardiovasc Imaging 2005;21(1):165–76.
18. McCollough CH, Primak AN, Braun N, et al. Strategies for reducing radiation dose in CT. Radiol Clin North Am 2009;47(1):27–40.
19. Paul JF, Abada HT. Strategies for reduction of radiation dose in cardiac multislice CT. Eur Radiol 2007; 17(8):2028–37.
20. Anonymous. ACR practice guideline for diagnostic reference levels in medical x-ray imaging. 2006. Available at: http://www.acr.org/SecondaryMainMenuCategories/quality_safety/RadSafety/RadiationSafety/guideline-diagnostic-reference.aspx. Accessed March 12, 2009.
21. Gray JE, Archer BR, Butler PF, et al. Reference values for diagnostic radiology: application and impact. Radiology 2005;235(2):354–8.
22. Suleiman OH, Conway BJ, Quinn P, et al. Nationwide survey of fluoroscopy: radiation dose and image quality. Radiology 1997;203(2):471–6.
23. Van Unnik JG, Broerse JJ, Geleijns J, et al. Survey of CT techniques and absorbed dose in various Dutch hospitals. Br J Radiol 1997;70(832):367–71.
24. Bauhs JA, Vrieze TJ, Primak AN, et al. CT dosimetry: comparison of measurement techniques and devices. Radiographics 2008;28(1):245–53.
25. Morin RL, Gerber TC, McCollough CH. Radiation dose in computed tomography of the heart. Circulation 2003;107(6):917–22.
26. McCollough CH, Bruesewitz MR, Kofler JM Jr. CT dose reduction and dose management tools: overview of available options. Radiographics 2006; 26(2):503–12.
27. McCollough CH, Schueler BA. Calculation of effective dose. Med Phys 2000;27(5):828–37.
28. International Commission on Radiological Protection (ICRP). 1977 Recommendations of the International Commission on Radiological Protection (ICRP Publication 26). Ann ICRP 1977;1(3):1–53.
29. International Commission on Radiological Protection. 1990 Recommendations of the International Commission on Radiological Protection (ICRP Publication 26). Ann ICRP 1991;21:1–201.
30. International Commission on Radiological Protection. 2007 Recommendations of the International Commission on Radiological Protection (ICRP Publication 103). Ann ICRP 2007;37:1–332.
31. Shrimpton PC, Wall BF, Yoshizumi TT, et al. Effective dose and dose-length product in CT. Radiology 2009;250(2):604–5.
32. Martin CJ. Effective dose: how should it be applied to medical exposures? Br J Radiol 2007;80(956): 639–47.
33. McCollough CH. Dose in computed tomography: how to quantitate, how to reduce. Paper presented at: NCRP 43rd Annual Meeting: advances in Radiation Protection in Medicine, 2007; Arlington, VA.
34. Gerber TC, Kuzo RS, Karstaedt N, et al. Current results and new developments of coronary angiography with use of contrast-enhanced computed tomography of the heart. Mayo Clin Proc 2002;77(1):55–71.
35. Gerber TC, Stratmann BP, Kuzo RS, et al. Effect of acquisition technique on radiation dose and image quality in multidetector row computed tomography coronary angiography with submillimeter collimation. Invest Radiol 2005;40(8):556–63.
36. Hausleiter J, Meyer T, Hadamitzky M, et al. Radiation dose estimates from cardiac multislice computed tomography in daily practice: impact of different scanning protocols on effective dose estimates. Circulation 2006;113(10):1305–10.
37. Jakobs TF, Becker CR, Ohnesorge B, et al. Multislice helical CT of the heart with retrospective ECG gating: reduction of radiation exposure by

ECG-controlled tube current modulation. Eur Radiol 2002;12(5):1081–6.
38. Trabold T, Buchgeister M, Kuttner A, et al. Estimation of radiation exposure in 16-detector row computed tomography of the heart with retrospective ECG-gating. Rofo-Fortschritte auf dem Gebiet der Rontgenstrahlen und der Bildgebenden V 2003;175(8): 1051–5.
39. Sanz J, Rius T, Kuschnir P, et al. The importance of end-systole for optimal reconstruction protocol of coronary angiography with 16-slice multidetector computed tomography. Invest Radiol 2005;40(3):155–63.
40. Earls JP, Berman EL, Urban BA, et al. Prospectively gated transverse coronary CT angiography versus retrospectively gated helical technique: improved image quality and reduced radiation dose. Radiology 2008;246(3):742–53.
41. Earls JP. How to use a prospective gated technique for cardiac CT. J Cardiovasc Comput Tomogr 2009; 3(1):45–51.
42. Hausleiter J, Meyer T, Hermann F, et al. Estimated radiation dose associated with cardiac CT angiography. JAMA 2009;301(5):500–7.
43. Mettler F Jr, Huda W, Yoshizumi T, et al. A catalog of effective doses in radiology and nuclear medicine. Radiology 2008;248:254–63.
44. Bluemke DA, Achenbach S, Budoff M, et al. Noninvasive coronary artery imaging: magnetic resonance angiography and multidetector computed tomography angiography: a scientific statement from the American Heart Association Committee on Cardiovascular Imaging and Intervention of the Council on Cardiovascular Radiology and Intervention, and the Councils on Clinical Cardiology and Cardiovascular Disease in the Young. Circulation 2008;118(5):586–606.
45. Budoff MJ, Achenbach S, Blumenthal RS, et al. Assessment of coronary artery disease by cardiac computed tomography: a scientific statement from the American Heart Association Committee on Cardiovascular Imaging and Intervention, Council on Cardiovascular Radiology and Intervention, and Committee on Cardiac Imaging, Council on Clinical Cardiology. Circulation 2006;114(16):1761–91.
46. Hendel RC, Patel MR, Kramer CM, et al. ACCF/ACR/SCCT/SCMR/ASNC/NASCI/SCAI/SIR 2006 appropriateness criteria for cardiac computed tomography and cardiac magnetic resonance imaging: a report of the American College of Cardiology Foundation Quality Strategic Directions Committee Appropriateness Criteria Working Group, American College of Radiology, Society of Cardiovascular Computed Tomography, Society for Cardiovascular Magnetic Resonance, American Society of Nuclear Cardiology, North American Society for Cardiac Imaging, Society for Cardiovascular Angiography and Interventions, and Society of Interventional Radiology. J Am Coll Cardiol 2006;48(7):1475–97.

# Index

*Note:* Page numbers of article titles are in **boldface** type.




Cardiol Clin 27 (2009) 679–682
doi:10.1016/S0733-8651(09)00093-9
0733-8651/09/$ – see front matter

**D**



**E**

F



G



I



L



M



P



R

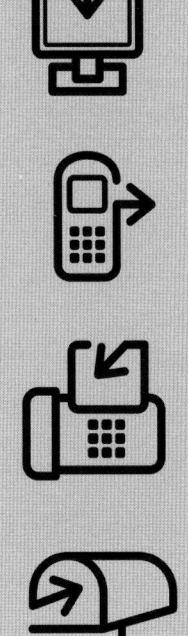

**United States Postal Service**

## Statement of Ownership, Management, and Circulation
## (All Periodicals Publications Except Requestor Publications)

| 1. Publication Title | 2. Publication Number | 3. Filing Date |
|---|---|---|
| Cardiology Clinics | 0 0 0 - 7 0 1 | 9/15/09 |
| **4. Issue Frequency** Feb, May, Aug, Nov | **5. Number of Issues Published Annually** 4 | **6. Annual Subscription Price** $244.00 |

7. Complete Mailing Address of Known Office of Publication (*Not printer*) (*Street, city, county, state, and ZIP+4®*)

Elsevier Inc.
360 Park Avenue South
New York, NY 10010-1710

Contact Person: Stephen Bushing
Telephone (Include area code): 215-239-3688

8. Complete Mailing Address of Headquarters or General Business Office of Publisher (*Not printer*)

Elsevier Inc., 360 Park Avenue South, New York, NY 10010-1710

9. Full Names and Complete Mailing Addresses of Publisher, Editor, and Managing Editor (*Do not leave blank*)

Publisher (*Name and complete mailing address*)

John Schrefer , Elsevier, Inc., 1600 John F. Kennedy Blvd. Suite 1800, Philadelphia, PA 19103-2899

Editor (*Name and complete mailing address*)

Barbara Cohen-Kligerman, Elsevier, Inc., 1600 John F. Kennedy Blvd. Suite 1800, Philadelphia, PA 19103-2899

Managing Editor (*Name and complete mailing address*)

Catherine Bewick, Elsevier, Inc., 1600 John F. Kennedy Blvd. Suite 1800, Philadelphia, PA 19103-2899

10. Owner (*Do not leave blank. If the publication is owned by a corporation, give the name and address of the corporation immediately followed by the names and addresses of all stockholders owning or holding 1 percent or more of the total amount of stock. If not owned by a corporation, give the names and addresses of the individual owners. If owned by a partnership or other unincorporated firm, give its name and address as well as those of each individual owner. If the publication is published by a nonprofit organization, give its name and address.*)

| Full Name | Complete Mailing Address |
|---|---|
| Wholly owned subsidiary of | 4520 East-West Highway |
| Reed/Elsevier, US holdings | Bethesda, MD 20814 |

11. Known Bondholders, Mortgagees, and Other Security Holders Owning or Holding 1 Percent or More of Total Amount of Bonds, Mortgages, or Other Securities. If none, check box → ☐ None

| Full Name | Complete Mailing Address |
|---|---|
| N/A | |

12. Tax Status (*For completion by nonprofit organizations authorized to mail at nonprofit rates*) (*Check one*)
The purpose, function, and nonprofit status of this organization and the exempt status for federal income tax purposes:
☐ Has Not Changed During Preceding 12 Months
☐ Has Changed During Preceding 12 Months (*Publisher must submit explanation of change with this statement*)

PS Form 3526, September 2007 (Page 1 of 3 (Instructions Page 3)) PSN 7530-01-000-9931 **PRIVACY NOTICE**: See our Privacy policy in www.usps.com

13. Publication Title: Cardiology Clinics
14. Issue Date for Circulation Data Below: May 2009

| 15. Extent and Nature of Circulation | | | Average No. Copies Each Issue During Preceding 12 Months | No. Copies of Single Issue Published Nearest to Filing Date |
|---|---|---|---|---|
| a. Total Number of Copies (*Net press run*) | | | 1975 | 1900 |
| b. Paid Circulation (By Mail and Outside the Mail) | (1) | Mailed Outside-County Paid Subscriptions Stated on PS Form 3541. (*Include paid distribution above nominal rate, advertiser's proof copies, and exchange copies*) | 814 | 715 |
| | (2) | Mailed In-County Paid Subscriptions Stated on PS Form 3541 (*Include paid distribution above nominal rate, advertiser's proof copies, and exchange copies*) | | |
| | (3) | Paid Distribution Outside the Mails Including Sales Through Dealers and Carriers, Street Vendors, Counter Sales, and Other Paid Distribution Outside USPS® | 394 | 337 |
| | (4) | Paid Distribution by Other Classes Mailed Through the USPS (e.g. First-Class Mail®) | | |
| c. Total Paid Distribution (*Sum of 15b (1), (2), (3), and (4)*) | | | 1208 | 1052 |
| d. Free or Nominal Rate Distribution (By Mail and Outside the Mail) | (1) | Free or Nominal Rate Outside-County Copies Included on PS Form 3541 | 99 | 114 |
| | (2) | Free or Nominal Rate In-County Copies Included on PS Form 3541 | | |
| | (3) | Free or Nominal Rate Copies Mailed at Other Classes Through the USPS (e.g. First-Class Mail) | | |
| | (4) | Free or Nominal Rate Distribution Outside the Mail (Carriers or other means) | | |
| e. Total Free or Nominal Rate Distribution (Sum of 15d (1), (2), (3) and (4) | | | 99 | 114 |
| f. Total Distribution (Sum of 15c and 15e) | | | 1307 | 1166 |
| g. Copies not Distributed (See instructions to publishers #4 (page #3)) | | | 668 | 734 |
| h. Total (Sum of 15f and g) | | | 1975 | 1900 |
| i. Percent Paid (15c divided by 15f times 100) | | | 92.43% | 90.22% |

16. Publication of Statement of Ownership

If the publication is a general publication, publication of this statement is required. Will be printed in the **November 2009** issue of this publication. — Publication not required

17. Signature and Title of Editor, Publisher, Business Manager, or Owner

Jean Fanucci – Executive Director of Subscription Services — Date: September 15, 2009

I certify that all information furnished on this form is true and complete. I understand that anyone who furnishes false or misleading information on this form or who omits material or information requested on the form may be subject to criminal sanctions (including fines and imprisonment) and/or civil sanctions (including civil penalties).

PS Form 3526, September 2007 (Page 2 of 3)